"If you're looking for a fitness solution that you can actually live with, this is your answer. Cathy Moxley has created a system that is practical and realistic for the novice, the avid exerciser, and every mom in between." –Carrie Myers Smith, President of Women in Wellness™ and author of *Squeezing Your Size 14 Self Into a Size 6 World*

"Cathy Moxley brings alive many of the amazing and undisputed benefits of physical activity. Her facts are right on target, and her entertaining and persuasive style will no doubt make a difference in the lives of many moms." –Leonard A. Wisneski, MD

"Busy moms will find a refreshingly different approach to fitness in Cathy Moxley's book. She has created a framework that takes into account one's readiness to embark on a new fitness plan, and delivers helpful tools, options, and insight for each stage of the journey to a fit lifestyle." –James O. Prochaska, Ph.D., author and internationally recognized developer of the stage model of behavior change

"Cathy Moxley is an experienced coach who doesn't just show you how to adopt a fit lifestyle; she takes you by the hand and guides you through the maze of everyday challenges to make your fitness intentions a lifelong reality." –Margaret Moore, Founder & CEO of Wellcoaches® Corporation

"This book is packed with plenty of "gems" including inspirational stories and practical tips from real moms who are achieving their fitness goals. If you're a busy mom looking to improve your health, you owe it to yourself to read this book." –Jerry Hill, CSCS, Owner, FitForce Camp, Philadelphia, PA, www.fitforcecamp.com

"Cathy's passion for fitness and her desire to help busy moms comes through in every line. If you want to exercise but don't know where to begin, this is the book for you." –Lissa Michalak, certified personal trainer and creator of BellyCore, New York, NY, www.trainwithlissa.com

"Cathy Moxley knows fitness and she knows busy moms. This book is a must-read for moms who want the benefits of fitness for a lifetime." –Scott Colby, President, SC Fitness, Inc., www.womensfitnesscamp.com

Real Moms Love Cathy's Book

"With Cathy's expertise, positive energy, and enthusiasm, I've taken small steps that have added up to big results. I've lost weight, have more energy, and look the best I have in years!" –Shari Greber, mother of two

"The tips in The Busy Mom's Ultimate Fitness Guide *really work. I am not kidding. I have been making huge strides in my exercise but also have put ME back on the priority list. Thanks, Cathy. This is truly life-altering stuff!"* –Nicolette Levchenko, mother of three

"I couldn't put this book down! It's an easy-read that's both funny and full of valuable information at the same time. Cathy gets her points across and sounds like she's having a conversation with you in your living room while she's doing it!" –Dotty Raleigh, mother of two

"If you're looking for the ultimate fitness solution, Cathy Moxley has it. She never fails to motivate clients and readers to set and reach big goals. Cathy walks her talk, understands the challenges busy moms face, and tailors fitness advice to their unique needs. If you want to discover the ultimate fitness solution once and for all, read this book." –Leslie McAlpine Hamp, mother of two, www.forwardmomentum.biz

THE Busy Mom's ULTIMATE FITNESS GUIDE

Get Motivated and Find the Solution That Works for You!

Cathy Moxley, M.A.

FitnessInSight™

Published by Fitness InSight™
13402 Queenstown Lane
Germantown, MD 20874
www.fitness-insight.com

ISBN-10: 0-9767800-0-3
ISBN-13: 978-0-9767800-0-7
Library of Congress Control Number: 2005933383

Book Design by Janice M. Phelps
Front Cover Photography by Amy Masser
Printed in the United States of America

This book is dedicated to my husband John, and our three children, Jenna, Jeff, and Matthew. You mean everything to me and I am thankful for our happy home!

This book is also dedicated to my own busy mom who always told me that I could do anything I put my mind to. I believed her because for as long as I can remember, she's been able to do anything that she put her mind to.

No one else can do this for you. It's up to you!
Congratulations on taking the first step!

Acknowledgments

I would not have been able to write and publish this book without the incredible support of my family. My wonderful husband, John has always believed in me and supported everything I do. During the writing and production of this book, he willingly took on many additional household responsibilities in order to give me the time I needed in the evenings and on the weekends to make this book a reality. My children, Jenna, Jeff, and Matthew were also great sports through the entire process and followed through on promises to fuel me with lots of hugs and kisses whenever I looked tired or grumpy in front of the computer.

I'd like to thank long-standing clients Kim Cohen, Linda Evans, Shari Greber, Stephanie Long, Kay Nash, Carol and Kelly Renshaw, Nicole Shannon, Valerie Singleton, and Tracy Zito. You are all an inspiration! When I think of successful exercisers who have made it work, I think of you. It has been an honor to walk along with you as you have built fitness into your lives — for keeps. What a gift you have given yourselves and your families!

There are also many other neighbors, family members, friends, clients, and women who attend my exercise classes who offered much encouragement as well as suggestions during the writing of this book. They shared their greatest fitness needs and struggles, as well as their ideas. Hardly a day would go by that someone didn't ask, "How's the book coming?" I never felt alone in this process. Thank you for believing in me and in the value of this book. I'd like to thank my parents, John and Concetta Schulien, my parents-in-law Judy Stolz and Ken and Madeline Moxley, Amie Cogan, Susan Joseph, Elisha Ehnes, Gee Lingberg, Tracy Vogel, Beth O'Connell, Kris Stuber, Syndy Kucner, Kelley Goehrung, Alyce Menton, Tracy Ritter, Laura Lowery, Jen Laubach, Brenda Moxley, Maria Selwood, Katie Valentine, Lisa Vogan, Katie Stiles, Terri Johnson, and many others. The Marriott Fitness Facility has been a constant in my professional life for many years and I owe much to the support and friendship of Dan Kolar as well as the rest of the staff and members. I'd also like to thank the many women who took the time to write and send me their stories for the section of the book entitled "Words of Wisdom from Busy Moms Who Are Making It Work." No doubt their real life stories will inspire you and spark some ideas for how you can make exercise fit into your own life.

Thanks go out to my business mastermind group – Scott Colby, Lissa Michalak, Jerry Hill, and Rex Laughlin for their support throughout the writing and production of this book. Each of these successful fitness entrepreneurs has been an invaluable resource for brainstorming, advice, and encouragement. Thanks to Ryan Lee, Jim Labadie, and Debbie Happy Cohen, whose business guidance has greatly inspired me. It was during their fitness business mentorship program that I decided now was the time to write "my book" once and for all.

I've got to thank Michael Port and Mitch Meyerson, who developed the Product Factory – an amazing environment that provided the support and accountability I needed to complete the entire first draft of this book during an intense twelve-week period. My Product Factory team leader, Leslie Hamp, my team buddy Jenny Lovins, Peggy Murrah, and the rest of my team "The Producers" were a constant source of help and encouragement.

I'd like to thank Amy Masser of Baby Face Photography for doing a great job with the cover photo shoot. She was incredibly patient with the kids and was able to get just the right shot. Also,

I'd like to thank Ron Roby of Roby's Photoshop for his painstaking, after-hours assistance editing and formatting all of the photos for the book. I owe deep gratitude to Phil Geyer of Harvest Moon Design for his amazing help with my websites and other technical needs. I would be nowhere without his expertise and advice.

When it came time to get outside feedback on the book's content and layout, there were many respected professionals, as well as busy moms who generously gave their time and thoughtful insight to make this book the best it could be. I was humbled by the care and detail that each of them put into their review of the book in progress — the professionals: Wayne Westcott, Ph.D., James O. Prochaska, Ph.D., Leonard A. Wisneski, M.D., Jeff Burruglio of Evolve Sports Medicine Group, Margaret Moore, CEO of Wellcoaches®, Carrie Myers Smith of Women in Wellness™, Sheila Watkins of Healthy Moms®, certified fitness professionals Meg Goodwin and Sharon Kolar, and the busy moms: Lorraine Branson, Julie Butler, Peggy Murrah, Dotty Raleigh, Cathy Schulien, Concetta Schulien, and Nicole Whitman.

Very special thanks go to my fabulous book editor and designer, Janice Phelps, for helping me bring this book to life! Her guidance has been invaluable and I am very grateful.

Lastly, I must thank God as the source of strength and all blessings in my life.

Table of Contents

Section One

Mind Games: Getting Motivated and Getting Ready

Section Two

Fitness Facts Every Busy Mom Should Know

Section Three

The Busy Mom's Exercise Levels

Section Four

A Busy Mom's Call to Action

Appendices

• SECTION ONE •

Mind Games: Getting Motivated and Getting Ready

Chapter 1

Information . . . Motivation . . . Solution

The Busy Mom's Experience

Moms have special fitness needs. Whether you are a new mom who wants to get your body back, or an old pro who needs to do something for *yourself,* time is an issue, as you well know. With those adorable, yet exhausting little people counting on you twenty-four hours a day, seven days a week, one thing you are sorely lacking is time to yourself. You certainly don't have the luxury of spending hours at the gym. Then there's the priority issue. Because your life revolves around taking care of other people, you probably tend to put your own needs pretty low on the priority list. Am I right? Maybe you're dealing with an inner struggle of how to use your child's naptime. (The to-do list always takes longer than the nap, and if you use that time for exercise, when will you get anything else done?) If you have school-age kids, you know all too well that the extra juggling involved in getting them to their activities divides the day into impossibly small pieces that seem to prevent you from getting anything accomplished.

As a busy mom with three kids myself, I know what it's like to try to fit exercise and other healthy habits into an impossibly filled schedule that usually leaves Mom's needs at the bottom of the list. On top of your family responsibilities, if you are also working outside of the home, balance can seem that much farther out of grasp. Once you get home from work, there's still dinner to think about, clean up, homework, baths, and a stack of mail and permission slips or a little laundry to go through before you can collapase. I once saw a comic strip where the husband was looking at the wife's calendar on the fridge (there were scribbles and notes on every date: doctor appt. 9 A.M., take the dog to the groomer 11 A.M., parent–teacher conference 4 P.M., sew patch on Brownie vest, pick up snack for soccer game, etc., etc., etc.). The husband commented, "Even the president isn't this busy!" The wife answered nonchalantly "Of course not . . . he's not a mom!"

Despite the chaos, smart moms know that if you don't take care of yourself, sooner or later, there won't be enough of you left to take care of everything and everyone else. You've undoubtedly heard this before, but have you taken that message to heart yet? If you're like a lot of moms, it *"sounds good,"* but there are a thousand reasons why you haven't done it yet.

Why now?

Hopefully, by picking up this book, you've decided that now is the time to finally put yourself on the priority list. Or, you definitely *want* to put yourself on the priority list and are hoping this book will give you the strategies you need to make it happen. Either way, congratulations! You're on the verge of living your life with more vibrancy and pride because you are doing the right things for yourself, in addition to your loved ones. This is a "get-your-act-together" book for every mom who has ever felt that leading a healthy lifestyle (i.e. getting fit, eating right, losing weight, managing stress, feeling balanced . . . you name it!) was out of her grasp. Maybe you've tried and failed too many times before, or maybe you've already categorized yourself as a non-exerciser or a fitness dropout. Maybe it all seemed too overwhelming given your daily responsibilities and a distinct lack of motivation. *Let's stop the whirlwind for a minute, take a deep breath, and figure this out . . . together.*

Information and Motivation

What can you expect from ***The Busy Mom's Ultimate Fitness Guide***? The purpose of this book is two-fold: First, I'll show you step by step how you can fit fitness into your life. I'll provide filtering for all of the information (and misinformation) out there. After all, with all the conflicting things you read, the diet industry hype, and all the infomercials, it's a wonder we're not completely overwhelmed into apathy. I'll cover the top tips in fitness so that you can get the most bang for your buck since time is at a premium. I'll also cover the practical aspects of how to fit these tips into your busy life. You'll learn fascinating physiological explanations on why these strategies make a difference. You may find out that when you have a grasp on the why, your motivation grows and things start falling into place. You may have heard before that fitness doesn't have to be all or nothing. But I'll go one step further: I'll show you the things that will make a difference along a wide-ranging continuum of *"bare minimum"* to *"Maybe I'll do a couple more things"* to a comprehensive exercise routine. You'll be able to choose the exercise plan that is right for *you*, complete with back-up plans and room for increasing and decreasing your routine as your needs change.

The second and even more important purpose of this book is to help you find the motivation necessary to be successful. You *can* do this! Many of you have been around the block before and may be saying, *"I know what I need to do . . . I just can't seem to do it!"* Don't worry — I won't be telling you what you should do in a perfect world. Even with a perfect exercise routine, life has a way of getting in the way. Instead, I'm going to shine a light on the common obstacles busy moms share and take my best shot at problem solving with you. It's my job to know what you are thinking, head off your objections at the pass, and share with you my enthusiasm for fitting in fitness! You'll receive encouragement and coaching to help you figure out what will make this time different for *you*. You'll learn how you can take small steps to start gaining the amazing benefits of fitness and feel more in control of this aspect of your life.

Finding Your Solution: What will make "this time" different?

At the crux of this book is one question. *What will make this time different from all of the other times you've tried to make fitness a part of your life?* We'll keep circling back to this important question throughout the book because herein lies the missing link for many people, the key to maintaining a fitness plan that works.

Only you can provide the answer to "What will make this time different?" But I can give you food for thought and a framework for the thought process. The end result will be finding what I call "Your Solution." Your solution is individual to you. It's not a one-size-fits-all plan, and it may or may not be traditional. What it will be is a fitness plan that is fluid, flexible, and works for you and your lifestyle.

Let's Get Started

Isn't it time you took charge of your health and wellness? It doesn't matter where you are now or how great or small your ultimate aspirations are, you can improve your health and well being. Don't wait another day! ***The Busy Mom's Ultimate Fitness Guide*** will help you map out a plan that will work to get you in shape and feeling great! It will provide the practical tips as well as the motivational encouragement you need to move yourself and your health up on the priority list. When you look at where the time goes in a typical week, chances are that doing for others seeps into every nook and cranny. If you don't speak up and stake your claim to a few time slots per week, the kids, hubby, school, work, volunteer committees, etc. will most definitely have ideas of how you could be spending that time. I'm fairly certain that with the responsibilities you have in your life, nobody else can or will help you set aside this time for yourself and your health and fitness needs. Nobody can do this for you except *you!* You have too much to gain and too much at stake to wait another day. Are you ready to absorb all the wonderful benefits awaiting you on this journey?

Chapter 2

If Exercise Came in a Pill

Imagine for a moment that there is a pill that has the following magical properties:

- ✔ Lowers your risk of heart disease, cancer, and diabetes
- ✔ Increases your bone density, thereby decreasing your risk of osteoporosis
- ✔ Conditions your heart and your lungs
- ✔ Strengthens your muscles
- ✔ Increases your metabolism
- ✔ Improves your flexibility
- ✔ Raises your HDL cholesterol (which is the good kind that you want to increase)
- ✔ Reduces back pain
- ✔ Relieves stress and depression
- ✔ Improves your blood pressure
- ✔ Helps you sleep better
- ✔ Improves your mental skills
- ✔ Helps you lose weight

Would you like this pill?

Do I hear a resounding *YES!*

It must be because it's hard to imagine someone not wanting this medication!

Just a minute, though — there's a catch . . .

This pill is only dispensed in single daily doses, meaning you can't get a big bottle to last you all month. You must get each daily dose individually each day, and if taken as prescribed, the results are *virtually guaranteed*. (Take another look at the list of results noted to remind yourself of all that you have to gain if you take this pill.) The "pill store" is close by, but it is in a pedestrian-only zone, closed to cars and buses. It's about a half-mile away, meaning that you'll need to walk about ten minutes to get there and another ten minutes back home.

It's time to take a third look at the list of benefits of this magic pill while I ask, "Would you do it?" Would you take twenty minutes out of your day to go get your daily dose if the results were *virtually guaranteed?*

Hmmm....

What's your answer? Still yes?

What if I told you that the pill I was dispensing was completely inert — just a placebo, and, in fact, it was the daily twenty-minute walk that delivers the benefits, rather than the pill?

Surprised?

A little disappointed?

Many of us have an easier time believing in a pill than in the capabilities of our own bodies . . .

The sad fact is that many of us have an easier time believing in a pill than in the capabilities of our own bodies. We are much more likely to put faith in the listed outcomes of a medication than in the movement of our own bodies, which we have control over. The truth is that exercise is the closest thing to a magic pill. Being active lowers your chance of developing some thirty diseases and troublesome medical conditions. This magic pill is not ginko biloba, not chromium picolinate, not vitamin C or any of the other products you see on the shelves of the supplement store, yet people flock to supplements in their continual search for that one, magic pill that will make a difference.

Exercise is the single best thing you can do to invest in your health.

I am here to tell you that a magic pill is indeed available and it is called *exercise*. Let's take a fourth look at that list of benefits:

- Lowers your risk of heart disease, cancer, and diabetes
- Increases your bone density, thereby decreasing your risk of osteoporosis
- Conditions your heart, lungs, and blood vessels
- Strengthens and firms your muscles
- Increases your metabolism
- Improves your flexibility
- Raises your HDL (good) cholesterol
- Reduces back pain
- Relieves stress and depression
- Improves your blood pressure
- Helps you sleep better
- Improves your mental skills
- Helps you lose weight

. . . And this is the short list! Check out Appendix 5 for "64 Reasons to Exercise" and refer to it whenever you need a little motivation. There truly are sixty-four (at least!) reasons to exercise. Exercise is arguably the single best thing you can do to invest in your health — delivering more health benefits than any other single health habit adjustment (except quitting smoking, if you are a smoker). While smoking is the leading cause of preventable deaths in the United States, obesity is the second leading cause, and the positive impact of exercise on obesity is well known. (*Sidenote to smokers:* You have much to gain from decreasing your smoking even if you aren't ready to totally quit!)

Did it sink in? Let me repeat it again, because taking this message to heart is the first step in gaining the benefits of fitness. Exercise is arguably the *single* best thing you can do to invest in your health — delivering more health benefits on its own than any other single health habit change. You can do lots of things that benefit your health in different ways, large and small — things such as eating more fruits and vegetables, using sunscreen regularly, or reducing your salt or sugar intake. In fact, I recommend doing all of the above to make a difference in some aspect of your health. However, none of those things, nor any other single thing you can do (except for our earlier caveat about quitting smoking) will have as many and as far-reaching health benefits in as many categories as E-X-E-R-C-I-S-E — moving your body!

Chapter 3

It's a Hard Pill to Swallow

So, if exercise really is the magic pill, why the heck aren't we all exercising regularly?

Why don't we have a humongous fitness boom on our hands and a culture of physical activity? Despite the proven benefits of exercise, more than half of American adults are not getting enough exercise to improve their health. Statistics show that only 12% of Americans belong to a health club of some kind, and this speaks nothing of how many actually *use* their memberships! Our children aren't faring any better. Only two states have mandatory physical education in public schools — Illinois and New Jersey, in case you were wondering. The effects are showing, literally, as we are a nation of growing girth.

The World We Live in Makes It Tough to Be Healthy

No one said this was going to be easy. The American obsession with weight loss is at an all-time high. You can't open a magazine or turn on the TV without encountering yet another product or program guaranteed to help you lose weight. There are pills, potions, packaged foods, books, videos, classes, websites, and gurus. Lots of people are making a lot of money, but are we getting anywhere?

Not likely.

America is as fat as ever . . . and getting fatter every year — meaning that the percentage of Americans in the "clinically obese" category has increased every year in the last twenty years. Let's take a look at an on-going study by the Centers for Disease Control (CDC), which compares the percent of each state's population who are considered clinically obese. In 1991:

- 4 states had the highest obesity rate, 15–19%.
- The remaining 46 states' obesity rates were below 15%.

Let's fast forward to the 2003 statistics:

- All 50 states had obesity rates 15–19% or higher.
- 31 states had obesity rates of 20–24%.
- 4 states had obesity rates greater than 25%!

What could be causing this epidemic?

Let's begin with some commonplace habits today that would have had Americans of an earlier era scratching their heads.

Think about the prevalence and accessibility of packaged junk foods. Yes, we had corn chips and cheese curls twenty years ago. If you wanted them with your lunch, Mom put a few in a little baggie to pack in your lunch box with your sandwich and apple. That was too much trouble, so the manufacturers started pre-packaging chips of every variety into single serving bags, which still wasn't convenient enough. Now, they come in plastic snack bottles presumably to make them even easier to eat!

Pizza used to be crust, topped with sauce and then cheese. Going hog-wild might include extra cheese or pepperoni. Now we've discovered that there's no reason to limit the cheese to lying on *top* of the pizza! You can buy a pizza with extra cheese injected into the outer crust and also sandwiched between two crusts like a layer cake! Think next about potato chips and chocolate — two delectable, yet distinctly different sinful treats . . . until recently. Today, you can buy chocolate in the shape of a potato chip! Go figure!

When do we eat and what are we doing when we eat? In times gone past, we ate at the dinner table, while conversing with family or friends. Today, the majority of meals for many people are consumed on the run, in a restaurant, in the car, or in front of the TV. We are often numb while we shovel food mindlessly into our mouths.

Super Size Syndrome

	20 years ago	Today
Bagel:	140 calories (3-inch)	350 calories (6-inch)
Cheeseburger:	350 calories	590 calories
French fries:	210 calories (2.4 oz.)	610 calories (6.9 oz.)
Soda:	85 calories (6.5 oz.)	210 calories (20 oz.)

Next, let's think about the "super size syndrome." Envision the hamburger, salad, soda, or cookie of the 1950s. Now think of the size of the hamburger, salad, soda, or cookie you'd purchase today. Chances are they are at least twice the size! What used to be the large is now the small, and the large has been replaced with the extra-large. Picture the sodas (or the coffees, for that matter) that you see coming out of your neighborhood convenience store. Surely they are no different than if you had put a straw into a half-gallon jug! And the more we get used to these serving sizes, the more it becomes second nature to overconsume. Ask friends who come from another culture and they will tell you that they have never seen a culture as, (ahem) . . . piggy, as Americans! We eat, and eat . . . and then we eat some more! For all the talking we do about low fat, low carb, diet this, and diet that, as a nation, we simply do not put our money where our mouths are.

Our activity habits are no better for the most part. Generations ago, many Americans performed daily tasks that involved physical work – milking cows, plowing fields, or working in a factory. Today, most people live very sedentary lives. Oftentimes we sit all day whether it's at home, at work, or in the car. Our culture and the very infrastructure of most towns and cities, especially in suburbia, rely heavily upon cars. Schools, shopping, and housing are no longer within walking distance in many communities as in days gone by. Many of us drive everywhere. Whether our destination is close or far, we hop in the car and go. Visiting our European and Asian counterparts, we would be stunned to witness their habit of walking and biking throughout their daily travels — physical activity built into their day.

Lifestyle-related health risks account for 51% of all deaths in the U.S.

Then there is the time factor. Time is king. First there was mail, then fax, then email, then email from our mobile phones. The pace of our lives has increased to the point that we expect instant results from everything that we do. There's instant oatmeal, online shopping, and phone banking. I'm sure you can think of even more examples. We're spoiled by instant gratification, as well. Ages ago, stores had something called lay-away. The customer would put a little money toward an item each week until they could finally afford the entire cost and get to bring the prized possession home. There's no waiting for what we want now. We put it on a credit card, we bring it home immediately, and we worry about the debt later. It's no wonder we expect our diet or exercise attempts to yield instant results, as well.

We are paying a dear price for our fast-paced lives and most of us don't even know it. We've slowly spoiled ourselves to the point where we avoid physical exertion at all costs. How many remote controls do you have in your household? Three? Six? Nine? I'll go first. We've got nine, I think: three TV remotes, one each for the VCR, DVD, digital cable, gas fireplace, and stereo, and then there's the garage door opener. Can you even imagine *not* having a TV remote control? There's self-propelled vacuum cleaners and drive-thru just about anything. We email co-workers instead of walking down the hall to speak to them in person. We rush around in the morning to get in our cars and sit . . . we scurry

Obesity is the second leading cause of preventable deaths in this country.

Cost of obesity-related medical treatment? $100,000,000,000

quickly into work and sit . . . we circle and circle for the closest spot at the mall, and we make good use of elevators, escalators, and moving sidewalks at the airport. Many of us simply do not move our bodies unless absolutely necessary!

The health risks associated with our lifestyle — inactivity, poor nutrition, obesity, and smoking, now account for 51% of all deaths in the United States. Smoking is still the number one killer in America — 435,000 deaths per year. Obesity is the second leading cause of preventable deaths in this country, with the last count at 26,000. How about the economic cost of obesity? One hundred billion dollars will be spent on the medical treatment of diseases caused by obesity, in addition to 65 billion dollars spent by consumers on the diet industry! Despite the money being spent, 95% of all diets fail!

The Individual Laundry List

Even though we live in a culture of inactivity, there still exists the opportunity to make our own decisions. What are the most common reasons why busy moms don't exercise? See if any of the below sound familiar:

Reasons Why I Don't Exercise

- I don't have time.
- I'm too tired.
- It's too boring.
- It's too hard.
- I don't need it.
- I'm too old.
- I don't have any equipment.
- It's too expensive.
- I don't need to lose weight.
- I've got a bad _____. [back, knees, etc]
- I don't like to sweat.
- It's not convenient.
- Nobody will go with me.
- I want to exercise in general, but I never feel like exercising!

The list could go on and on. Because fitness coaching is what I do for a living, I've heard all the reasons:

"By the time I (fill in the blank) and (fill in the blank), there's really no time for exercise."

"You wouldn't believe the number of emails I had to return, and then I've got to pick up the dog from the groomer, and then..."

After a while, they all start to sound a little bit like "the dog ate my homework," and I find myself walking a tightrope between two positions:

a) nodding sympathetically about all the stresses and scheduling challenges that prevent one from exercising regularly and . . .

b) the tough-love approach that says, "If it was a priority, you would make time, period."

Let's look at two examples.

Meet "Gary," a single, 28-year old man who is a computer programmer and belongs to a health club he never visits. Gary finds himself working late night after night and declares that he is just too busy to make time to get to the gym. Then . . . one of those times he is at the gym, he meets an attractive woman he would like to know better. Lo and behold . . . he suddenly starts getting out of work earlier and finds himself being able to make it to the gym on a regular basis.

Now, let's look at "Irene," a married, 57-year old woman, who has never made much time for fitness. She leads a full life and can't imagine donning exercise clothes on a regular basis. It's just not part of who she is — until she has a heart attack. Suddenly, she has exercise appointments three times per week . . . under close supervision at a cardiac rehabilitation facility. Not exactly the circumstances anyone would want as a motivator to exercise.

Did the dog eat your homework?

If you were told that you had a life-threatening disease and that you would die if you didn't exercise for twenty minutes three times per week, every week you'd find time to do it, wouldn't you? Of course you would. *The bottom line is that we all have time for the things we make time for.* We find time or make time for those things that are most important to us and for the things that have become habits.

Think about the many things that you feel you have to do. It's a busy morning and you are trying to get the kids out of the door for the school bus. You're running short on time, so you....send little Johnny on his way without making his lunch? No. That's not negotiable. Little Johnny's lunch has to be made, right? You make sure it gets done. (Well, maybe you could just tell him to buy his lunch that day, so maybe that's not a good example!) Here's another: Everybody does laundry (at least eventually) because you have to have clothes to wear. You have to shower, brush your teeth, and dress before you leave the house (I hope). These things are not negotiable. You just do them. Why is exercise *not* in that category? Think about this point. For example, if I'm not going anywhere special, blow-drying my hair and applying make-up are negotiable. I'll do it if I have time after my workout. But my workout is not negotiable. What makes something go into the non-negotiable, must-do category in your mind?

To do:

- ❒ Bake cake
- ❒ Balance checkbook
- ❒ Haircut
- ❒ Return shoes
- ❒ Plan party
- ❒ PTA
- ❒ Vaccinations
- ❒ Vet appt.
- ❒ Dry cleaners
- ❒ Homework
- ❒ File taxes
- ❒ Plant bulbs
- ❒ Call repairman
- ✔ Exercise

Priority and Habit

Priority and habit: There you have it. Take a hard look at your reasons for not exercising and be honest with yourself about the priorities in your life. If exercise is not a priority for you, hopefully it will become one by the time you finish reading this book. The first step is admitting where it falls on your priority list right now rather than rationalizing about your reasons for not exercising regularly. The reasons are certainly real, but they are not insurmountable when exercise is a priority. We'll look at solving them together.

How does something (like exercise) magically move up the priority list? Think about our examples of Gary and Irene and the simple ratio of pros vs. cons. The cons are your reasons why you can't exercise (time, inconvenience, etc.). These reasons certainly do exist, and may overshadow the pros when you only have 4 or 5 pros or reasons why you should exercise. Once your list of pros grows to **50**, for example, the cons will pale in comparison to all that you have to gain. We'll discuss using pros and cons in more detail in the next chapter as a part of your "Toolkit to Get Your Mind on Track." In the mean time, to build up your own list of pros, why not take another look at Appendix 5: 64 Reasons to Exercise?

The Stages of Change

Have you been beating yourself up because you aren't doing something (anything) that you know you should be doing? Maybe it's nightly flossing, or keeping your bills organized, or yes, exercising regularly. Whatever it is, you feel guilty because you think you should be doing it, cut and dry, simple as that. Research shows, however, that making a personal change is not as simple as "just do it" (with all due respect to Nike), and it's not operated like an on-off switch. Rather, I'd like to teach you about a wonderfully comforting framework that explains how all behavior change is a *process* that goes through five well-defined stages. I call it "wonderfully comforting" because you'll feel like an incredible weight has been lifted off your shoulders as you abolish the guilt of not-yet-taking action on whatever the goal is. The "Stages of Change" developed by the renowned psychologist Dr. James Prochaska can be applied to any health-improvement topic, such as quitting smoking, eating healthier, or beginning an exercise program. The Stages of Change deal with your psychological readiness to tackle this change. The stages are progressive, which means that you don't skip stages. Whether you go through them quickly, slowly, or even get stuck in a stage, the goal is always to get to the next stage. The goal is not always action. The goal is not automatically to change the behavior, but simply get to the next stage in your *readiness* to change the behavior. Can you see the difference?

While we go through the Stages of Change, we will continue to refer to good old-fashioned pros and cons in our quest to figure out where you are in your ability to change. Let's take a look at the five stages of change . . .

Stage 1

Precontemplation

"I can't." "I won't."

The goal: To start thinking about it.

If you are mentally in this stage for a certain health behavior change, you may not even think there is a problem, or you may know there is a problem but you think it's insurmountable. You have no intention of changing in the forseeable future. You may be uninformed or under-informed about the consequences of not changing a given behavior. Or you may have tried to change a number of times and become demoralized about your ability to do so.

I've got several busy mom friends and relatives (who shall remain nameless!) in this stage for exercise. I'm thinking of them right now. I'm fairly certain that these particular women don't exercise because they are naturally thin, although there are many other reasons to be in this stage. We've been brainwashed that the primary reason to exercise is to lose weight. And as busy moms, if you don't need to lose weight, there's no sense adding exercise to your already full to-do list. Unfortunately, all of the other fabulous health benefits are not given nearly the credit they deserve.

This stage usually means one of two things: "I can't" or "I won't." If you are feeling "I won't," you simply aren't interested and don't think there is a problem. The way to get to the next stage rests on learning more about the pros — the reasons why you'd want to make this change. Unfortunately, people in this stage tend to avoid reading, talking, or thinking about the issue at hand, and therefore won't be seeking out information about the reasons to change. Precontemplators typically underestimate the benefits of change and overestimate the costs, but are unaware that they are making these mistakes. And if you're unaware of your error in judgment, how can you change? Two major forces can help precontemplators to progress. The first is developmental events, such as a mid-life reevaluation of your lifestyle or a catastrophic event that can push you to the next level. The second is environmental events — the bombardment of messages from a variety of sources including loved ones and the media. Personalized, early intervention efforts from someone that cares can make all the difference.

If you are feeling *"I can't,"* you are aware of the need to change, but you think it's too complicated or too difficult. In order to get to the next stage, you need help overcoming the cons. You may be pessimistic or dejected, and could use lots of problem-solving information and encouragement to get to the next stage. Rest assured, you are probably not in precontemplation for fitness — because you are reading this book! You *want* to change this habit!

Double and then triple your list of pros so that it's much longer than your list of cons.

Stage 1 Contemplation

"I may."
The goal: To move from thinking to deciding

Contemplation is the stage in which someone intends to take action within the next six months. The *"I'm thinking about it"* stage is for those sitting on the fence. It's cognitive quicksand — the place many people GET STUCK! You want the benefits of change, but you aren't yet ready to make the sacrifices necessary, haven't figured out a way around the obstacles in your life, or maybe you just don't know where to begin. This balance between the costs and benefits can produce profound ambivalence. It all sounds good to you, but nothing really jumps out at you. This is the stage of *"I'm just not motivated. I really need to get motivated."* Can you hear the whiny tone of voice? You are not imagining it. There is often a lot of frustration and desperation in the contemplation stage. The reason why contemplation can be a chronic stage is that you just have not found a compelling reason to change. You may have a lot of reasons, but not *compelling* reasons. Your list may include all the stock reasons you should want to (fill in the blank), but you haven't taken any of them to heart.

> *Sandy is a self-described fitness wanna-be, otherwise known as a chronic contemplator. At times, she has exercised on and off, but for one reason or another, she cannot maintain the habit. Sandy feels terrible because she knows she "should" be exercising, but just hasn't been able to get going again. What is she to do?*

The goal when you are stuck in the contemplation phase is to gather more information, do more reading and even some soul searching to move from thinking to actually *deciding*. One of the best things you can do to get yourself to the preparation stage is to make a really thorough list of pros and cons. The pros are the things that are going to make this change worthwhile.

The cons are not necessarily what's bad about making this change, but rather what the obstacles are. There must be a pro that is strong enough to really get you going, to tip things in favor of going to the next stage. Or, if it's a con that's really holding you back, you need to resolve that issue in order to move forward.

Latch on to a particularly compelling benefit.

Stage 3

Preparation

"I will."
The goal: To do it!

Now we're getting really close. You're done thinking about it and weighing all the pros and cons of taking on this change. You intend to take action in the immediate future. You have begun figuring out exactly what is going to work for you and you are trying to get to the next stage — action! When you are in the preparation stage, what's going to help you is developing concrete plans and setting up strategies to meet your goal. If exercising more regularly is the goal, you might be calling around to different health clubs to see what their specials are, or you're looking into personal trainers in your area, or you are looking at your weekly calendar to decide when you are going to schedule your workouts.

When Stephanie first called me, she was definitely in preparation mode. She had been thinking about beginning an exercise program for a while and decided to take the plunge after looking at my website. She liked the fact that we were going to look at the big picture when designing her exercise routine — how we could set her up for success over the long term. In fact, once she got rolling, she applied the same preparation principles to many other areas of her life — organizing her work habits, family calendar, and countless other things she had been meaning to do for herself. What a success story!

In preparation, you should be setting up your plan . . . but also your back-up plan. When you consider all of the options available to you, you must seriously consider how realistic each one is. (A vow to begin an early morning fitness routine is doomed if you're the type that hits the snooze alarm a dozen times.) When you plan well — for real life, not for "in a perfect world," you're much more likely to end up with a plan that you can stick with. Be honest with yourself about what you can see yourself doing, what's going to trip you up, and how you're going to handle those situations.

Give careful consideration to how realistic each option is for you, when formulating your fitness plan.

Stage 4

Action

"I am."

The goal: To keep doing it!

Actually doing it is great! After all the thinking and planning, it feels good to finally be here and taking action. So how's it going? Are things working out as you thought they would? The first six months of a behavior change is a fragile period, with the highest risk of relapse during this time. Establishing a new habit is hard! (I don't think you needed me to tell you that!) It takes a lot of time and commitment. You've got to work out the kinks and get yourself used to your new routine. If something happens to throw you off track (illness, a business trip, the holidays), you might have a hard time staying consistent because the habit isn't ingrained yet.

Alyce is a great example of action. She was ready, she was determined, and she was organized. It wasn't easy, and I know it's still not easy for her. She works full-time and comes home to the same things many of you do — dinner, baths, and homework. Yet, by planning each week's work-outs ahead of time, putting them on her calendar, and following through with personal training appointments, we have been able to set small goals week by week, creating a plan that is really happening! She's losing weight, feeling great, and thrilled with her accomplishments!

This is the time when support and accountability can really make a difference. If you are going it alone and you hit a snag, there's no one around (besides that little voice in your head) telling you to pick yourself up and get back to it. We tend to ignore that little voice so it's really nice when someone else cares about your goals besides you! You want to make sure a little blip doesn't turn into a complete relapse. Having a partner, a buddy, or a coach during this fragile period will allow you to encounter all of the normal obstacles with support. You'll be able to solve problems together and then, when the same obstacles appear later when you are on your own, you'll know what to do.

Support and accountability can make all the difference.

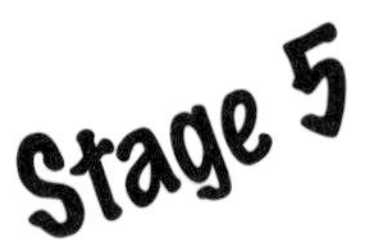

Maintenance

"I still am."
The goal: To stay here, with no danger of stopping.

If you've been doing a new habit for over six months now, congratulations! This is considered the maintenance stage of a behavior change. Maintenance occurs when the behavior has become a habit and is maintained over time. Your job now is to be wary of boredom and make sure you don't gradually slip back into your old ways. You become increasingly confident that you can sustain the change and the risk of relapse decreases more and more over time.

Shari has been working out with me for over two years. She is a vibrant, upbeat, working mother of two. Her boys are five and two and her job is demanding, to say the least. Shari is always up for whatever is coming her way — she always gets the job done, and after that she can be found cleaning out the garage or volunteering at a homeless shelter. Shari was also eating take-out seven nights a week and not exercising. I guess something had to give! Shari decided it was time to find a way to fit exercise into her busy life. She had tried home exercise; she had tried joining a gym. Nothing stuck. She and I started working out together twice a week. I got Shari started on a running program and lifting weights. Now, despite being arguably busier than many of my other clients, she is the most consistent. She just never misses her appointments. Even when she's short on time, she'll fit in part of it, or she'll always reschedule to another day. We've gradually figured out a way she can make a decent dinner for her family more often than not — thanks to just a little advance planning and a crock-pot. As for the running . . . a while back I suggested we run in a 2-mile race together. She didn't think she could do it . . . but she did. Then there were a couple of 5Ks (3.1 miles) this past summer . . . and she thought those were FUN but just about her limit. That was a few months ago. She called me the other day asking about an ad she saw for an upcoming 10K race (6.2 miles)! Did I forget to mention that she's dropped two dress sizes along the way?

Support can be just as important during maintenance as during the beginning stages of action. If you are feeling bored, you might want to look into ways you could vary your routine. Maybe you'd like to train for one of those charity walks, or try out an exercise class you've never done before, or schedule a few visits with a personal trainer to perk up your routine. Keep it up and way to go!

Keep it fun and varied so you don't get bored.

How Should I Use This Information?

Understanding the stages of change is a great start to finding your fitness solution. You get to stop feeling guilty that you haven't taken action yet, when, in fact, you might not have been ready to take action. The first step in applying this information is to identify what stage you are in and recognize that *your only possible goal is to get to the next stage in your readiness to change.* Your goal is not to take action unless you are truly in the preparation stage already. Remember that you can be in different stages for different habits. You may be "thinking about it" for exercise, but taking "action" for healthy eating, for example.

This book includes strategies for all of the stages of change. Section One of this book should be very helpful for the pre-contemplation and contemplation phases. It focuses on increasing the pros, decreasing the cons, problem solving and getting over the mental hurdles of deciding to make a change. Section Two takes you to the next level — preparation, laying out the components that are necessary for a well-balanced exercise routine and other considerations to help you set up a concrete plan that is best for you. Section Three is all about action. You will select the plan that is best for you and give it a shot! Section Four is perfect for maintenance, containing supportive information for how to maintain your habit and your commitment for the long haul.

Now that we have looked at all of the reasons why you might not have figured out your fitness solution yet, let's move on to helping you move forward!

Let's Review:

Stage 1: Precontemplation

- ★ The goal: *To start thinking about it.*
- ★ Tip: Build up the list of pros to far outweigh the cons.

Stage 2: Contemplation

- ★ The goal: *To move from thinking to deciding.*
- ★ Tip: Latch on to a compelling benefit.

Stage 3: Preparation

- ★ The goal: *To do it!*
- ★ Tip: Formulate a plan with small steps.

Stage 4: Action

- ★ The goal: *To keep doing it!*
- ★ Tip: Seek support and accountability.

Stage 5: Maintenance

- ★ The goal: *To get to the point where there's no danger of stopping.*
- ★ Tip: Keep it fun and varied.

Chapter 4

A Toolkit to Get Your Mind On Track

This is still Section One so we are still focusing on your mind . . . not your body! It's time to negotiate yourself through the mental mine field of priority, habit, and mind games.

How can we get our minds on track to get our bodies moving and our expectations realistic? Having the right mindset is crucial to your success in finding your fitness solution. We are going to address the important business of getting rid of your mental baggage, fixing your mindset, and looking at your fitness commitment from a philosophical point of view that will keep you nourished for the long-term. It's a real mental workout, so let's dig in!

Your toolkit includes:

1. Getting Rid of the Baggage — Unhealthy Mindsets
2. Accepting Ownership and Admitting Priorities
3. Taking a Break to Take Stock
4. Creating a Vision and Setting Goals
5. Weighing the Costs vs. Benefits
6. Knowing Thyself — Preferences and Personality
7. Anticipating and Strategizing around Obstacles
8. Finding a Common Thread
9. The "Click" Factor
10. Practical Keys to Making It Work
11. Supportive Philosophical Musings — It's All in the Attitude

Remind yourself that more may be better than less, but some is definitely better than none.

Getting your workout in, even if it's not your whole routine, is valuable for fostering continuity, which is just as important as the fitness benefits of the exercise.

Bottom line: Habit is more important than content.

Getting Rid of the Baggage — Unhealthy Mindsets

Do you have an unhealthy mindset that is undermining your ability to feel good and be successful? The most common unhealthy mindsets are all-or-none thinking, pessimism, stereotyping, and the mighty quick fix.

All or None

Are you under the impression that it's full-throttle workout or bust? Many of us have heard the recommendations, read the "most effective exercises" for this, that, or the other . . . and feel obligated to do it a certain way or — well — *"It's not worth it . . . I might as well not do it at all."* Am I right? The truth is, there are many health benefits to be gained from even modest amounts of exercise. Have you ever skipped a workout when you thought it'd take too long? Think again. When you don't have time for your full routine, a shorter one will do! Too often, an all-or-none mentality robs us of the Holy Grail of exercise — consistency! Consistency is, in my opinion, the most important part of exercise. Would you believe that content is completely secondary? "Why?" you ask. Let's just say that I have met with countless clients or potential clients throughout the years who want me to design the perfect routine that will give them the body beautiful that they so desire. The point that I need to gently get across to them is, "I can design it, but that doesn't mean you can do it, or that you will do it long enough to see the results." Their response may include a bit of dejection or denial. What good is the perfect routine if you can only stick to it for exactly five weeks?

Wouldn't it be much better to start with a more modest, realistic exercise routine that really whets your appetite and that you can build on?

Or, maybe you have a full-fledged routine that you do when you have time, but you also have mini-exercise options for those busy weeks that serve a great purpose — *keeping you feeling on track*. Ask yourself, "What's realistic today . . . this week . . . in general?" What's "good enough?" There are plenty of days that good enough truly is good enough — a victory — a true success! Maybe your normal routine is 45 minutes of cardio and a 30-minute weight training routine. On a day when you are tired or pressed for time, wouldn't it be better to do a quick 20 minutes on the treadmill and then some crunches rather than doing nothing at all? You betcha! Do not let perfectionism ruin your opportunity to get some kind of workout in.

With my personal training clients, each client has good days and bad. Sometimes you can predict them — hadn't had much sleep the night before, it was a stressful day at work, etc. Other days, there's really no explanation. You just don't feel your best or your strongest. You just have the blahs during your workout. Some clients feel disappointed in themselves that they didn't have a great workout that day. I try to reassure them that for consistent exercisers, that's *okay*. Some workouts were meant to serve no other purpose than to maintain a consistent habit. It wasn't great, it wasn't pretty, but you did it. It served a valuable purpose of maintaining continuity and holding the status quo for your fitness level. So what if you didn't make great gains that day? Fall into the trap of canceling workouts altogether whenever you don't feel quite up to it and you start down a slippery slope!

Pessimism

Have you tried and failed before? Started and stopped a dozen times? Convinced that you won't ever . . . get fit, lose weight, etc.? Often times, we are our own opponent in mental mind games. Think of how you would speak to a close friend who was struggling with how to make a certain lifestyle change and kept faltering. Would you berate your friend? Or would you

There is no such thing as a crash course on your wellness journey.

offer consolation and encouragement? Be a good friend to yourself and give yourself the gift of faith, understanding, and a second (or third or fourth) chance. You can do this! You are going to get the right information, cultivate the right expectations, and do *something* to improve your health! Do not give up!

Stereotypes and Self-consciousness

Stereotypes in fitness are everywhere. Unfortunately, we are subjected to body-image baggage and athletic-ability baggage that can take the wind out of our sails with one look at the local health club's newspaper ad. Contrary to some images, already being fit, looking good in exercise clothes, or having been athletic or coordinated in high school are not prerequisites for exercising! Fitness is for everybody . . . but more importantly, it's for every *body*. Your body needs to move and you shouldn't let anybody or anything make you feel like you are not good enough, or coordinated enough, or fit enough to do *something*. There are a huge variety of fitness options now available to women beyond the glitzy, "everybody is staring at you" type of clubs. Family-friendly clubs and down-to-earth all-women clubs abound. Community centers have homey fitness centers and there is much you can do in the comfort of your own home.

For most of us, however, it's not a problem of other people stereotyping us. Rather, we've done it to ourselves! Are you guilty of categorizing *yourself* as a non-exerciser, a confirmed couch potato, or a lost cause? Have you declared that you don't *need* exercise because you don't need to lose weight? Even if exercise clothes and health clubs are not for you, there is much you can do for your health. Research has shown that even a modest increase in physical activity can have a significant impact on your health. A mere 30 minutes or more of movement per day can decrease your risk of heart disease and a host of other ailments. The most important thing is finding something you enjoy and getting started!

The Quick Fix

Are you truly ready to stop looking for a quick fix? Can you truly accept that it doesn't exist? Can you accept your body as it is *today?* Can you free yourself from using your body to measure your self worth? Can you recognize that your body deserves to be respected and cared for, not judged? Are you ready to negotiate how much you are willing to give (in terms of diet and exercise changes) and accept what your body (given your genetics) is willing to do with that level of change? Everyone is different, and your exercise and nutrition plan needs to be realistic for your life, your whole life, in order to work. The best plan means nothing if you can't stick with it. Try making one small change, then another, then another. Make the behavior the goal, not the result. Things have a way of building on one another.

You must abandon the search, the quest, the *longing* for the quick fix. This is so important, I feel the need to say it again.

Read the following sentence aloud, slowly, giving emphasis to each word:

"I must abandon the search, the quest, the longing for the quick fix."

I know it's hard. We *really* want to believe it can happen. We are eternally hopeful, faithfully clinging to the possibility that there's an easy way to do this. We perk up our ears and open up our wallets with every new infomercial, pill, and potion. The temptation is all around us and will never go away. As long as there are people who want to lose weight, there will be people trying to sell them a quick fix. They know our weakness and will prey on it! Just say no! There is no such thing as a crash course on your wellness journey. Looking toward a deadline or a finish line almost always comes with a rebound effect. You know those diets that prescribe a fairly stringent program while you lose weight and then propose a maintenance plan that is less stringent to keep it off? Those plans always set off a red flag for me. I believe the body takes a certain amount of time to reach equilibrium for any given set of eating and exercise habits. When your habits change (for better or for worse), your body slowly readjusts to those habits — maybe up a few pounds or down a few pounds.

A better way is to plan to continue doing whatever you did to lose weight in order to keep it off. When you make a few changes, ask yourself, *"Can I see myself doing this forever?"* If so, keep it up and see if you're able to reach your goals with that level of lifestyle change. If the results aren't enough for your desires, ask yourself if you're willing to make a few more stringent changes forever and see what results that brings. Slow and steady wins the race. I have a Nike poster hanging in my exercise room that shows a woman sitting on a weight bench wiping her brow. The slogan under the photograph reads, "There is no finish line." Some people may think that's depressing. I feel quite the opposite. It reminds me every day, that this is not a race, that I'm in this for the long haul, and that I'm just enjoying the ride with no intention of stopping.

I have a neighbor who once commented to me that he'd "sign up" if I could promise him that he would lose twenty pounds in a month. I smiled and went into my usual speech about how if he was still looking for a "quick fix," he wasn't ready to work with me yet. This neighbor is savvy in finances and my husband, who was there at the time, later suggested that I use the analogy of a 401(k) plan vs. a get-rich-quick scheme as a metaphor for different approaches to fitness. I thought it was brilliant! Exercise is indeed like putting money into a 401(k) . . . it's an investment that you make on a regular basis that pays off in the long run. Looking for a quick fix for weight loss is just like looking for a get-rich-quick scheme — it rarely works. Furthermore, the longer you put off starting your 401(k) plan, the less time you have for the money to compound, and, therefore, you have less total money to show for your investment. Do you really want to start and stop a half-dozen get-rich (a.k.a. get-thin) schemes? The likely result will find you no better off in the long run. Isn't it so much better to start a reasonable approach, one that can be working consistently for the rest of your life?

Where do you invest your money — in a 401(k) plan or a get-rich-quick scheme?

And so it is with fitness.

You must abandon the search, the quest,
*the **longing** for the quick fix.*

Did you see yourself in any of these menacing mindsets? It's hard to change your thinking overnight, but you can start replacing some of those ingrained messages and put yourself on the right track.

Accepting Ownership and Admitting Priorities

Important vs. Urgent

I like to call this the message of "change it or quit complaining." Too harsh? We talked a lot about priorities in Chapter Three. We talked about the concept that exercise doesn't have to be full-blown and it doesn't have to take a lot of time. We posed the tough message that "If it was important to you, you'd do it . . . period." In order to move forward, you need to stop blaming other things for your stalled exercise habits. Accepting ownership means realizing that you are in control of your daily life and your decisions on how to spend your time. We all have twenty-four hours in a day, and it is up to us how we choose to spend them. Now, of course I know that you don't get to pick how to spend each and every hour of your day (don't we wish!). Some people definitely have more discretionary time than others. But, when we are honest with ourselves, we know that's not the real issue. The president of the United States exercises regularly, and I'll bet he's "busy." I know single moms who exercise regularly, and I know they are busy, too. Regardless of your busy-ness, exercise is one thing that you can't delegate! Rich or poor, busy or not, nobody can exercise for you! Accept ownership for that decision. Be honest with yourself about your priorities and decisions on how you spend your time. Put it on paper. Are you putting everyone else's needs above your own? Do you make sure you attend to everything you "owe" other people, but when it's something just for yourself, it's the first to go when things get busy? Think about your workouts from the point of view of "important" vs. "urgent." By now, you probably believe that exercise is *important*. The problem is that each individual exercise session will never be *urgent*, which is why it's so easy to blow off a particular workout. Keep in mind the notion that each workout is important from the standpoint of keeping you on track, in addition to the actual benefits of the exercise session. Also, start thinking about what this says from a self-esteem standpoint as well as the example you are setting for your children. You must take your own needs and put them on the priority list. And you must protect that time and treat an appointment with yourself with as much respect as an appointment with someone else. Are you telling yourself that you are less important than everyone else in your life? I hope not!

Finding Time vs. Making Time

Finding time and making time are both great tools for accepting ownership and admitting your priorities. What's the difference between the two?

> *Finding time* means keeping your eye out for little snippets of time that can make a big difference. Can you consolidate your errands or household chores? Get up early one day a week, carve out a midday chunk once a week, and commit to one exercise session every weekend? If so, that's one example of how you could exercise three times per week without undue changes on any one part of your schedule.
>
> *Making time* means examining your priorities and the things that are using up your time right now. Are there things that are taking up chunks of time that are not very fulfilling or valuable that you might want to cut out in order for you to make room for exercise? A little too much TV in the evenings, perhaps? Are there things you could delegate? Chores that the kids could help with?

Taking a Break to Take Stock

When you "take a break to take stock," you set aside some time to look at what is really going to make this time different from all of the other times you have tried to make a lifestyle change. It's not a quick look or a rushed and half-hearted completion of a checklist that's merely "one more thing you have to do." Rather, I am talking about a thought-provoking inquiry process that will crystallize where you are, where you want to go, and what it's going to take to get there. After all, how can you reach your goals if you haven't taken the time to put them into words and formulate a plan? You may be nodding in agreement, but busy moms have a habit of cutting corners on themselves and on prep work. Resist the urge to merely read through this section. You are the best expert at what is going to work in your life. Invest in yourself, block off some time on your calendar and actually do the exercises. You will be so glad you did. Use Appendix 1, *"Charting Your Course"* to organize your thoughts and make a commitment to yourself on paper.

Fitness and Wellness Coaching

One of the best ways to take stock is with a fitness or wellness coach. You may not have heard of fitness or wellness coaching, but it is a growing field and may soon be as commonplace as personal fitness trainers! This book is, in effect, coaching you to find your fitness solution. Sports coaches bring the best out of athletes, business coaches bring the best out of executives, and a fitness or wellness coach brings the best out of your efforts to lead a healthier life. A personal trainer will focus on the specific content of your exercise session. A coach will focus on everything else it takes to make fitness a part of your life. A coach will help you set goals and will hold you accountable to your goals. Think about other areas of your life for which you have outside accountability. When there is a deadline at work, you may need to be accountable to a boss or a client. At home, you are certainly accountable to your family for the things they need from you. People are counting on you to produce a report, get dinner on the table, or pick up a birthday present. Does anyone really care (besides you) whether or not you get your workout in or whether or not you follow your eating plan this week? Because of the lack of outside accountability, we don't often place a high enough priority on these things that are indeed important to us. A coach fills this gap. A coach will encourage you, problem solve with you, and provide a systematic framework for all the health and fitness habits that you usually do on your own. And rather than just taking things as they come, a coach will take a pro-active approach to help you anticipate, strategize, and work through obstacles and challenges that threaten to throw you off track.

Fitness and Wellness Coaching Can Make "This Time" Different

If you're like a lot of moms, you've been dreaming of looking or feeling a certain way for a long time, but something else always takes precedence.

Why continue to go it alone (and continue to get nowhere) when you could have someone in your corner supporting you?

Wouldn't it feel great to get there, once and for all?

I like to compare a fitness coach to a round-the-clock personal trainer because your coach will be concerned with a lot more than just what happens during the few hours a week that you are together. You'll feel supported and know that someone else is there to help you every step of the way, just as you are for so many people in your life. If you want to know more about coaching, visit me at www.fitness-insight.com. You can also visit www.wellcoaches.com. Wellcoaches® is the leading organization for fitness and wellness coaches. Check them out!

My client Tracy was an out-of-shape and overwhelmed stay-at-home mother of three — a 4-year-old daughter and 8-month old twins. Her husband works nights and sleeps during the day and is unable to help much with the kids. When we first started working together, Tracy thought she would never be able to fit in exercise or get a handle on a nasty stress-induced cookie dough habit. She never had a break from the kids and food seemed to be her only source of enjoyment. The first thing Tracy and I did in our coaching relationship was define her wellness vision — what it would look like and feel like to be at her best. We talked a lot about what would motivate her and what would be the biggest obstacles. When we set her first week's goals, Tracy was surprised that they were so small. But the next week, and then the next week, things began to grow. We'd gradually add in just a little exercise where she could. Not that there weren't slip-ups. I think the positive nature of the coaching relationship helped Tracy see that minor setbacks were not the end of the world and that she could continue onward. Tracy was thrilled and surprised that by the end of twelve weeks, she was not only taking regular walks with the babies, but found herself craving them. The food-obsession had all but disappeared, and she had lost six pounds to boot! She couldn't believe that what had seemed like such small changes each week had added up to so much by the end of twelve weeks. She's still at it, slowly but surely!

Creating a Vision and Setting Goals

Your Vision

What does being healthy and fit mean to you? What does it look like? What does it feel like? What do you see in your mind when you picture your "goal self" with regards to health and fitness? Where do you see yourself in one year? Five years? Are there certain things that you are doing regularly, ways you are feeling on a scale of one to ten? Why settle for floating adrift when you can chart a course for your health and fitness journey . . . and it is indeed a journey. Businesses have vision statements that encapsulate their long-range aspirations; you can do the same. Putting some thought into several well-selected sentences can help give you a sense of what you are striving to become. There are no right or wrong answers with your personal vision. The statements are meant to be very general, but possibly unique descriptors of what represents your longer-term goals, desired outcomes, habits, feelings, and motivators. Your overall wellness vision might address lots more than just fitness — it might touch upon stress, nutrition, sleep habits or leisure and relaxation. It might also include references to your overall values, life goals, and relationships.

Here are three examples of vision statements (with permission) from wonderful women for whom I have much admiration. Notice the difference in tone for each of these different women. All three of these amazing ladies have made great strides in their health and well-being:

> *I will gain back control of my life, to look better and feel better about the person I am, the person looking back at me in the mirror every day. I am a priority and have a place on the daily and weekly priorities in my life. I will make myself a priority every day and make time to focus on me only. Exercise is a big part of this as it is a stress reducer. I feel better when I exercise and can face the "daily routine" with great strides, patience and a positive attitude. My actions, as a result, will impact the people around me, especially my girls. By watching*

their mother they will have a role model in regards to a healthy lifestyle.

I want to make up for lost time and both feel and look young, slim, and sexy while I am still in my 30s. I want to be "bitten by the fitness bug" — having internal motivation and commitment to exercise on my own in addition to with my personal trainer.

I am a healthy, relaxed, fit woman with lots of energy to do all the things I want and need to accomplish for myself, my family, and my community. I look good, feel good and set a good example of healthy living for my children. I take care of myself by making good habits a top priority — eating healthy amounts of nutritious foods, exercising vigorously at least three times per week, staying smoke-free, and being attentive to my spiritual self. When I face obstacles or feel tempted to backslide into old negative habits, I will remind myself of my many reasons for wanting to be healthy. I will also remember the love of my Creator, and thus feel a strengthening of my commitment to good stewardship of the life that has been gifted to me.

Powerful stuff, isn't it? Did you get a smile on your face just reading these vision statements? Did you feel the energy, the commitment, and the certainty of self? Imagine how much more of an impact it would have on you if you were reading about yourself. Giving thoughtful consideration to what you really want for yourself and putting it down on paper makes it more real and that much more attainable. Your vision provides a compass for your personal wellness journey and both acknowledges and honors all the best things inside of you that are just waiting to get out! Take some time, write your vision statement and post it where you can be reminded of it when you need a boost. You'll be glad you did!

Goal Setting

Goal setting is very important. You've heard it before: If you don't know where you are going, how will you know when you get there? Goal setting fixes the problem of feeling adrift and vague in your fitness and wellness aspirations. But make sure you do it the SMART way. S-M-A-R-T is the common acronym for effective goal setting: specific, measurable, action-oriented, realistic and time-sensitive. Take a look at each of those words one at a time. Are your goals SMART?

Specific, as opposed to vague.

Measurable, as opposed to not quantifiable.

Action-oriented, as opposed to *"kinda," "sorta," "when I get around to it."*

Realistic, as opposed to pie-in-the-sky.

Time-sensitive, as opposed to "one of these days."

Which of the following two goals sound SMARTer?

- *"My goal is to get in shape and eat better."*
- *"My goal is to exercise three times per week every week — twenty minutes of cardio plus a mini weight training routine and to stop eating leftovers off the kids' plates."*

Three months is the most common time frame used for long-term goal setting. That amount of time is long enough to see real results, but short enough that you can't just forget about them. The next step would be to break down some shorter-term goals, possibly weekly, that will feed into achieving your three-month goals. Whatever time frames you choose, the most important thing is to make sure your goals are written down, visibly placed somewhere, and accountable to someone other than yourself or the cat.

Weighing the Costs and Benefits

Weighing the costs and benefits is no different than making a detailed and thoughtful listing of *pros* and *cons*. Remember, the most important predictors of success have to do with balancing out the pros and cons, the costs and benefits, and the motivators and obstacles. Or more specifically, in order to move forward, the pros (benefits) have to outweigh the cons (obstacles). It sounds like common sense, but oftentimes we simply aren't honest with ourselves. If you do not have a *compelling* motivator or if you don't have an effective strategy to deal with a significant obstacle, you will not be able to succeed. Let's take a closer look:

The Pros = The Benefits = The Motivators

Ask yourself: *Why do I want to change this behavior? What do I have to gain?* Why is this important to me? What is going to be so great when this is changed? What would be so bad if I never changed this behavior? Answer these questions and just write! Make the list as long as possible and don't hold back. Include the short and silly reasons, as well as the serious and heart-felt. How many have you come up with? Do you have any really strong, compelling motivators? In order to be successful your list of pros needs to be longer than your list of cons. In addition, you will need strong motivators to exist, they will need to be tangible and somewhat immediate-feeling, and you will need to keep reminding yourself of what they are.

Motivators for adopting a healthier lifestyle might include:

- ❒ Feeling less stressed and more in control
- ❒ Feeling less self-conscious in a bathing suit
- ❒ Being able to wear all the clothes hanging in your closet
- ❒ Having a healthy atmosphere in your household and setting a good example for your kids
- ❒ Taking pride in doing something for yourself
- ❒ Reducing your risk of early-onset heart disease that runs in your family

What does your list look like? Which items really speak to you and are compelling enough to make you *act?*

The Cons = The Costs = The Obstacles

Ask yourself: Why shouldn't I change this behavior? What's too hard about this? What's going to get in the way? Why haven't I succeeded before? These may seem like trick questions. The word "cons" might throw you off because there's no real downside to exercise and getting healthier, right? What you should really be focusing on are the costs — the obstacles. Think about your laundry list for what's getting in the way and list it out. Next, we'll get to brainstorming and problem-solving one by one.

Know Thyself — Preferences and Personality

While you are deep in thought about what your goals, motivators, and obstacles are, it's a good time to think about your preferences and personality. Are you someone who likes to have alone time when you exercise or do you crave a fun, social atmosphere? That might mean the difference between joining an exercise class vs. taking walks on your own. Do you prefer variety and get bored easily or are you most successful when you have a structured, predictable workout that you don't have to think about? When is your energy level highest? Are you an early morning person or a night owl? Do you like to chop things up into small, manageable bites or "get it all over with?" Do you get overwhelmed easily or do you prefer to dive into new things? All of these factors will impact your success level. Don't fool yourself. Remember in goal setting, the letter "R" stood for "realistic." Your fitness solution must fit your preferences and your personality.

Anticipate and Strategize around Obstacles

You should have a good-sized list of obstacles by this point for why you haven't yet found a workable fitness solution. We can't just leave that list unchallenged, now, can we? Ask yourself what it's going to take to accomplish your goals and how you'll handle the glitches that are bound to happen along the way. Most obstacles aren't insurmountable; they just require thoughtful strategizing and a commitment to stay the course despite a little drifting. No new habit is born overnight. And most obstacles do not appear overnight. Since most of your obstacles are indeed predictable, you can anticipate them and plan for how you will handle them. And you need practice handling them. Many fitness efforts fail because the "perfect case" scenario is the only situation you've planned for. How often does your week go exactly as planned? Not very often if it's anything like my household! Recall the section on all-or-none thinking. This is where it is applied. Be sure that you develop back-up plans and a "good enough" mindset for days when you need to stay on track, but can't do your normal routine.

So what's your favorite obstacle? Is it a crazy schedule? If so, one technique you could use is to look at your calendar every Sunday night, figure out when you can exercise that week and write it into the schedule. Is it "something always coming up"? That might mean you need to find a time of day when there's the least chance of interference, like early morning. Is motivation and accountability your weakness? You may need to plan exercise dates with a friend or a personal trainer.

Find a Common Thread To Stay on Track

I believe one of the most valuable factors that can contribute to your success, especially during the fragile beginning period, is *some kind of common thread that strings the weeks together to become months and then years of a sensible approach and a healthy lifestyle.* Remember, you're just living your life, in a healthier way, but slow and steady as she goes. You are not on a crash course to fitness and then you're done. Your common thread could be a personal trainer that you see at regular intervals (exactly how often may be determined by your budget), or a fitness/wellness coach. When I started my personal fitness training business, I decided to focus on short-term personal training. I reasoned that personal training should not be just for the wealthy, who could afford to have someone helping them on an ongoing basis. Rather, wouldn't it be great to help people with more limited budgets get started with the right information and let them continue on their own? As it turned out, most of my supposed short-term clients wanted to train on an ongoing basis. And it wasn't necessarily because we were doing exercises that they couldn't do on their own. It was the relationship. It still is the relationship. My clients know that I'm going to ask them about the workouts they were supposed to do on their own since I last saw them. They know that I care about their on-going healthy lifestyle. I have become their common thread. Working out with me, whether it's twice a week or twice a month, keeps things on track for them. Your common thread doesn't have to be a personal trainer or a coach, but it has to be *something*. Your common thread could be an exercise class if you've developed friendships and camaraderie there, or a neighbor or family member who is just as committed to this as you. Some of us have an old exercise buddy with whom we have a history of talking each other *out* of exercising or who cancels frequently. This person is *not* your common thread. Your common thread helps you stay the course over time. Your fitness level is defined by what your habits are at the time. You can't save it up. Keep up the habits and you keep that level of fitness. You keep that level of health. You keep that level of wellness and sanity!

Kay came to me this past spring just after the birth of her second child. She is a beautiful woman full of witty repartee and a twinkling smile. She was also about sixty pounds overweight at the time. Kay told no one that she was coming to see me. After all, she had gained and lost weight many times before. This time, Kay and I mapped out a plan in baby steps, for she knew all too well that she wouldn't stick to anything too restrictive. And with the amount of weight she wanted to lose, she would need to stick with the program for a while. For the eating side of things, we decided not to be too structured. We planned out what would be good choices for breakfasts, lunches, dinners, and snacks. The only rule we set was for her to keep a food diary that we'd review together every week. For exercise, Kay started out working out with me three times a week, and then gradually weaned herself to once a week exercising with me and doing the other workouts on her own. During the rough spots, Kay and I have even kept in touch with daily emails. Kay has often said that having someone in her corner has made all the difference. She's lost twenty-six pounds and counting!

The "Click" Factor

You know when something just goes click in your brain? For whatever reason, you've mentally turned a corner and you're ready to do things differently. It makes sense and you feel the energy and the commitment. You get it and there's no going back. Think back to those stages of change. The click may happen when you suddenly get a really compelling motivator to make a certain change. Sometimes it's a catastrophic event — a parent having a heart attack at a young age, a diagnosis of an illness like diabetes. Sometimes it's a doctor's appointment where the doctor tells you that "if you continue on this path . . . " The click could happen reading this book, it could happen when you see an old friend who has lost fifty pounds and is feeling on top of the world. The click sometimes comes a little more gradually before you know it happened. You may not know you have it until you have the flu and it occurs to you that you *miss* working out and can't wait to get back to the gym. You might be standing at the kitchen sink mentally going through your day and you realize getting in a workout is the first thing on your mind. You can't necessarily predict when it's going to happen, but you can continue to expose yourself to the positive messages and work towards your new healthy habits. Envision yourself already there and move toward it.

Practical Keys to Making It Work

You're still in planning mode, and it's time to take a quick look at a few considerations that really make a difference.

- **Fun** – Taking a walk can be blissful alone time. Taking an exercise class can be great social time. Bike riding with the kids can be great family time. What's going to be fun for you? Whatever it is . . . if it's not something you enjoy, no wonder you're not sticking to it. It doesn't have to be conventional, just move your body and have fun.
- **Convenience** – You've got enough stuff to do that isn't convenient. Why would you want to drive clear across town or fight rush hour if you don't have to? Take a good look at what would be convenient or you will never stick to it.
- **Plan it into your day** – Make your fitness routine just as much of a "given" as anything else on your to-do list. Plan specific days and times for your workouts.
- **Flexibility and a back-up plan** – Remember, a back-up plan and small ways to do "something" when you can't do your normal routine is key to keeping yourself active and on track. Business travel, a sick child, and deadlines at work can spell trouble unless you've already figured out what you'll do when obstacles arise.
- **Put it on your appointment calendar** and treat it like any other appointment.
- Once it's on your calendar, **protect its place on the schedule.** This goes back to the notion that fitness is important, but each individual exercise session is not urgent. Therefore, when something else comes up . . . do you quickly give up the workout? When you plan

exercise into your day, it must be with a fair amount of conviction. Yes, I keep talking about back-up plans and flexibility, but show a little respect to yourself and don't give up your appointment with yourself at the drop of a hat. When someone wants you to do something during the time you had planned to exercise, try saying "That time won't work." And then suggest an alternative. Tell them why or don't tell them why. The choice is yours. Just give it a try. It's probably an option more often than you think. Or how about just plain *no*?

Supportive Philosophical Musings — It's All in the Attitude

Staying in the right mindset is important. Our thoughts cause our feelings. Therefore, what you fill your brain with determines your mindset. Reading motivational books and articles, watching motivational programs, and seeking out positive role models all make a difference. How about what you say to yourself? Try to pay attention to your internal dialogue – the little voice that talks to you inside your head all day. Is it a positive voice or a negative voice? Attitude makes a big difference! Take a look at my free-flowing thoughts on fitness and a healthy outlook on personal wellness . . .

Cathy's Fitness Philosophy

*I believe that personal wellness is dynamic — that it is a journey, not a destination. It's figuring out what fits into your life at any given point — balancing the job of caring for the body you've been given with enjoying the life you've been given. I sometimes think that too many people put off feeling good about themselves until "after"...after they lose ten pounds, after they fit into a certain pair of jeans, after they stay on the "XYZ" diet successfully for "x" number of weeks. I believe in feeling good and accepting your body **now**, and then gradually taking small steps that don't cost much, but will add up in the long run. Most people who go that route find that the small successes motivate them to add more and bigger changes down the road. I always encourage clients to only make changes that they can see themselves still doing a year from now. Many people aren't ready for that approach though. After all, it goes against our natural tendency to seek the short-term payoff. We live in a society of immediate gratification and promises of quick fixes and instant results. But how many more times do you want to start, fall off and then restart that stringent eating and exercise routine, each time re-calculating the date by which you'll see a certain result if you start again "now"? Sadly enough, those poorly patched-together weeks fly by until it is a year later and you are in the same place as when you started. Why not take a different approach? Start with the long-term in mind from the beginning. What changes and habits can you incorporate into your life that you can see yourself doing . . . open-ended . . . just because you've decided "that's the way you live your life now"? Something has to click inside you to be ready. And when you're ready, you need support and continuity — a common thread of some kind that will help you stay the course through the weeks and months until you've found the part within you that will keep it going on your own. I believe in the power of taking charge of your life — reflecting on what you want your life to be and then making intentional choices. I believe in focusing on the habits and actions that build health, rather than focusing on the result. If you focus on enjoying today and enjoying the journey, you will see the results along the way.*

My Challenge to You is Attitude.

- ✔ This is a long-term process.
- ✔ It's a choice, a priority, and a lifestyle.
- ✔ You're ready to accept the fact that there are no quick fixes.
- ✔ You're done with extremes.
- ✔ It's about forever.
- ✔ There is no finish line.
- ✔ There is no hurry to arrive. There is no train to catch.
- ✔ It's all about making small changes little by little that you have no intention of ever stopping.
- ✔ You are building good health and fitness from the inside out.
- ✔ Strive for consistency, not perfection.
- ✔ Focus on the actions, not the outcomes.
- ✔ You will be giving yourself the gift of doing something good for yourself.
- ✔ Those small, good things will slowly add up.
- ✔ Time will pass and you will still be doing those things.
- ✔ Small health changes lead to bigger ones.
- ✔ The results *will* come. Do they really have to come within a pre-conceived time frame in order to have been worthwhile?
- ✔ Be positive, be easy on yourself, and treat yourself as a friend.
- ✔ Your needs are just as important as those needs you are meeting for other people. Have the self-esteem to keep your appointments with yourself just as you would with someone else.

✔ Keep in mind that you need to be ready to change before you can act.

✔ Just start and then just do.

✔ One day and one week at a time.

✔ You are positive, flexible, and resilient. Let it shine through!

✔ Avoid complaining about how you look (especially if you have daughters). Accept who and where you are now and move forward.

✔ Change your environment to set yourself up to succeed! Do not rely on "willpower" unequipped with the things you need to succeed and amidst a sea of temptations.

✔ "Fight the good fight." Make a good faith effort to practice habits that are as healthy as you're willing to sustain and then accept the outcome as what's meant to be.

✔ Stop comparing yourself to neighbors, friends, celebrities, or the people featured on weight-loss ads. Your body and your response to eating and exercise changes are unique to you.

• SECTION TWO •

Fitness Facts Every Busy Mom Should Know

Chapter 5

Fitness Basics: What and Why

Now that you've got the right mindset, let's talk in a little more detail about the amazing benefits of exercise. Understanding the wonderful things you have to gain . . . that you will gain . . . will do wonders in getting you committed to getting started! We'll tackle in detail the base knowledge that's important when you are building your fitness solution. After all, how can you make an educated decision about the nature and extent of your fitness efforts unless you know what is to be gained from all of the possibilities?

Aspirin or Pepto-Bismol? That is the question. That is the question that I often pose to new clients. Let's say you have a headache. It's a doozy. So you go to the medicine cabinet and you take out the Pepto-Bismol. You take a big swig of the pink stuff and – your headache doesn't go away! You figure you didn't take enough. Guess you better go back and take a double dose. What's the error here? What? Pepto-Bismol doesn't work for headaches? Ah-ha! No wonder your headache didn't go away. You were taking the wrong medicine for what was ailing you!

And so it is with fitness. It's a common mistake to have the wrong expectations about what benefits you can gain from each kind of exercise. A new client might complain to me, "I've been doing tons of crunches every day, and I can't seem to get rid of the fat on my stomach!" Unfortunately, that's no surprise.

Crunches are exercises that target the abdominal muscles, but do nothing for the *fat lying on top* of your abdominal muscles. Don't get me wrong. Crunches are a great exercise and they can definitely improve the appearance of your abdominal region. But they do so by making the stomach muscles tighter and firmer — which holds everything in a little better and thereby improves the look from the side-view, for example. Decreasing the fat lying on top of the abdominal muscles is another story. This is the myth of spot-reduction. You can't pick where you want to lose fat and do a certain exercise for that region. Fat loss is nonspecific, coming from wherever your body wants to release it. This happens when you burn more calories than you consume (through a variety of eating and exercise habits) with some help from Mother Nature. You can thank your parents or you can curse your parents, because genetics are the bottom line regarding where you store your fat. Some of us genetically store more fat in the abdominal region, others in the hip and thigh region. Wherever your trouble spot, it's stubborn for a reason!

5 Components of Fitness

So how do you develop the right kind of expectations? The first step is to get specific about your fitness goals. Often, my new clients will say they want to *"get in shape"* . . . which is great, but a little too vague to set up a plan. The best course of action is to learn the different components of fitness as well as what types of exercise affect each of those components. The following list is one commonly used method of specifying five distinct components of fitness. I've been known to get somewhat technical in my explanations, and I admit that I can get a little carried away. You won't hurt my feelings if you don't think it's as fascinating as I do, but do know that I'm going into such detail for a good reason. Knowing "why" and "how" all this stuff works can really help you take the fitness message to heart. You may just hear yourself saying, *"Wow. I never thought of it like that!"*

1. Cardiovascular Endurance/Aerobic Fitness

What It Is

Cardiovascular endurance is thought by many people to be the most important component of fitness. It's defined as the strength and efficiency of your heart, lungs, and blood vessels. How does all this work? Your heart is a big muscle with a hollow cavity inside. Each time your heart beats, the heart expands to fill with blood and then contracts to pump the blood out into the blood vessels. The oxygen and nutrient-rich blood is then carried to all the cells in your body through a complex network of smaller and smaller blood vessels. Whether you are fit or unfit, your body needs a certain amount of blood circulation to sit at rest, go about the business of your day, or to exercise. (The harder the activity, the more oxygen and therefore blood circulation is needed.) *How* your body delivers that amount of blood circulation is the question. If you are aerobically fit, your heart muscle is stronger and is therefore capable of stronger contractions. Each time your heart expands, it will fill with a greater amount of blood and is able to contract more strongly and deliver more blood with each heart beat. Therefore, your heart doesn't have to beat as often to deliver the same amount of blood circulation. Have you ever had your resting heart rate measured? You can do this yourself. Find your pulse and count it for a full minute while you are sitting at rest. This is called your *resting heart rate.* Average resting heart rate is about 72 beats per minute. A resting heart rate slower than that (in the sixties or even the fifties) signifies a strong heart that doesn't need to beat as many times per minute as compared to a less fit heart. A resting heart rate higher than 72 usually signifies a weaker heart that needs to beat more times to accomplish the same amount of work. Would you rather have a strong heart that delivers lots of blood with each beat or a weak little heart that needs to beat a lot of little times to deliver the same amount of blood?

Your well-conditioned heart and blood vessels go a long way in the prevention of heart disease and also in your capacity to comfortably participate in a variety of activities in your day-to-day life. I'm talking about whether or not you get winded if you have to run up a flight of stairs, need to sit down after running after your 2-year-old who's gotten loose, or feel completely drained after a day of shopping.

How To Improve It

There's only one way to improve cardiovascular endurance and that is through aerobic exercise, such as walking, jogging, biking, or step aerobics. When you use large muscle groups continuously for an extended period of time, your body requires more oxygen and blood. This increased demand forces your body to adapt and therefore grow and compensate for next time. The result is a stronger and more efficient heart!

2. Muscular Strength

What It Is

Muscular strength is the maximal amount of force that your muscles can generate once. This means that if something weighs a lot, can you lift it or not? Can you move that piece of furniture on your own or not? Can you pick up that huge box or not? In a health club setting, some real weight training enthusiasts (mostly men) test their muscular strength by measuring the maximum amount of weight they can lift once. Let's take the bench press as an example. They might add more and more weight to see what's the absolute highest weight they can do . . . if they only have to do one repetition. You, of course, don't have to measure your muscular strength that way. We all usually have a sense of how strong we are, especially when it comes time to pick up luggage or hoist a box onto a high shelf. Do you do these kinds of things yourself, or are you immediately looking for your hubby or someone else with muscles to help?

How To Improve It

The primary way to improve muscular strength is through some type of resistance training. This can be in the form of weight training with dumbbells, weight machines, or even elastic tubing or body weight exercises. The key, however, is that your muscles grow and adapt when you overload them. If the weight you use is not challenging, you will not get stronger. Improving muscular strength is specific to the muscle(s) that you work, meaning that you need to do specific exercises to hit each of the major muscle groups.

3. Muscular Endurance

What It Is

Muscular endurance is the ability of your muscles to exert a smaller level of force over an extended period of time. If muscular strength is defined by "Can you lift this huge box or not?," muscular endurance is defined by "How far can you carry the box?" Muscular strength and muscular endurance are really best thought of as points along a continuum of muscular work. When you lift really heavy weights very few times you are building mostly muscular strength. When you lift lighter weights many times, you are building mostly muscular endurance. Workout somewhere in the middle and you are getting a little of both components of fitness.

How To Improve It

Just as with muscular strength, muscular endurance is improved specifically based on what muscle groups you target. The primary way to improve muscular endurance is again through some type of resistance training — using weights, elastic tubing, or body weight exercises. You also build muscular endurance during aerobic exercise in the muscles that are primarily used for whatever the activity is. If you think about it, biking, for example, asks your leg muscles to contract over and over again for an extended period of time. Therefore, in addition to building cardiovascular endurance, you are also building muscular endurance for your leg muscles while you bike.

What about muscle "tone" and "firmness"?

These are the buzzwords you might commonly hear and they definitely paint a picture in your mind of what many of us want to achieve for our muscles! (You would not be alone if "how big of a box you can pick up and how far you can carry it" are secondary concerns for you!) What is muscle tone, anyway? Let's say you have 100,000 muscle cells in your quadriceps (thigh) muscles. Even when you are just sitting around, a certain percentage of those muscle cells are at least partially contracting. After all, if they weren't, you would be oozing out of your chair! If you have more muscle "tone" because these muscles are used to working out, a higher percentage of your muscles are partially contracted, even at rest, causing the muscle to be a little "firmer" in look and touch. Therefore, you improve muscle tone and firmness when you increase both muscular strength and endurance.

4. Flexibility

What It Is

Flexibility is the ability of your muscles to go through a full range of motion. There is definitely a genetic component based on subtle differences in muscle length and the specific site where your muscles attach to your bones. You probably didn't need me to tell you that. We all seem to know how flexible we are starting in childhood. Either you were one of the kids on the playground who could drop into the splits in ten seconds, or you were one of the kids staring with your jaw hanging down thinking "How'd she do that?" Even now, if ten busy moms were lined up and asked to touch their toes, they'd all be different and would all probably know ahead of time whether or not they'd be successful! Maximizing your genetic capacity for flexibility is especially important for those of us who aren't naturally very flexible. Increased flexibility helps keep your muscles limber and receptive to reaching and bending, and comfortably participating in a variety of activities. It can also be helpful for

Unfortunately, those who need to improve their flexibility the most usually avoid stretching, while the super-flexible do it in excess.

preventing injuries, such as pulled muscles. The theory is that when a muscle is used to going through a large range of motion, it will be able to better withstand a sudden, accidental increase in muscle length without pulling or tearing.

How To Improve It

Because there is a strong genetic component to flexibility, there's only so much you can do to improve it. That doesn't let you off the hook, though! Very few of us are maximizing our genetic potential. You *can* improve your flexibility as much as possible by doing stretching exercises. This is another component of fitness for which specificity matters. You don't improve "overall flexibility." Rather, you need to do specific stretching exercises for each muscle group that you would like to improve. Unfortunately, the people who need it the most typically avoid stretching because they *"aren't good at it"* and . . . *"It hurts!"* The Gumby-type women you see stretching up a storm on the mats in your local health club don't really need to be doing so much stretching because they are already so flexible.

5. Body Composition

What It Is

Body composition is the percentage of fat in your body compared to the percentage of muscle. The amount of fat on your body may not seem at first glance to belong in the same category as the other components of fitness. After all, it is not a "capacity" that you can train, like the other four components of fitness. It is, however, a marker of metabolic fitness — the efficiency of your body at managing the storage and usage of fat as fuel, and so it belongs. I'll bet you would like to increase your body's efficiency at *using* fat as fuel. (I can't say I've met as many busy moms who are desperate to increase their body's efficient *storage* of fat!)

Body composition is a much better indicator of obesity than the scale or height/weight charts. It is not uncommon for a small person to have a lot of fat on her body, just as it is not uncommon for a larger person to have a great deal of muscle. When you know your percent body fat, you truly know how much of your weight is fat vs. muscle and whether or not you are *overfat*, (a better term than overweight). Most people have heard that "muscle weighs more than fat," which is why two people who weigh the same amount, but have different body compositions can have very different shapes and even wear completely different clothing sizes. Pound for pound, muscle is firmer and more compact than fat, resulting in smaller circumference measurements and a smaller clothing size. Picture a wet towel (muscle) and a dry towel (fat) and envision scrunching each of them up into the smallest ball possible. Which one is smaller? The wet towel, of course. It's also hard as a rock and weighs more. The dry towel weighs less, but takes up more room and is soft and fluffy! Which would you rather have on your body? Something that is harder and smaller, even if it weighs a little more, or something that is soft and spacious yet weighs less?

Body composition can be measured by a number of different specialized tools, available at most gyms and through fitness trainers. Each method has a different degree of accuracy and it's best to only compare measurements against other measurements using the same tool and preferably with the same person doing the testing. Body composition measurement will be most meaningful if you think you are in an average to slightly overweight weight range. Many thin women actually have an unhealthy body fat level without even knowing it. It can also be valuable to measure your body composition in order to have something to compare to as your fitness improves. On the other hand, if you already recognize that you are significantly overweight, knowing your exact percent body fat is not that important, and may frustrate or upset you.

How To Improve It

Because body composition is expressed as the ratio of fat to muscle on your body, you can impact it from two angles. Isn't that great news? You can improve the percentage of fat on your body by decreasing your fat *and* by increasing your muscle mass. Unfortunately, as I already mentioned, you can't pick where you want to lose fat and there are no specific exercises you can do to lose fat from a specific area. You decrease fat on an overall basis by changing your diet and also through exercise. The goal is to decrease total fat and calorie intake so that intake is lower than the calories that you burn. You also impact body composition through exercise. Aerobic exercise burns a big chunk of calories during each workout and trains your body to burn calories more efficiently at rest and all throughout the day. Weight-training exercise increases muscle, which then increases metabolism thereby increasing total calories burned each day. On top of that, the increase in muscle directly impacts the ratio of fat to muscle. Isn't it great that there are so many ways to impact body composition? We will touch upon all of these mechanisms in detail throughout the next few chapters.

Moving On

Understanding the five components of fitness is step number one of your fitness knowledge base. You are now able to get a lot more specific about your goals, rather than declaring that you want to "get in shape." Step number two is to understand which kinds of exercise impact each of these five areas.

Components to Your Exercise Routine

- Aerobic Exercise
- Resistance Training
- Stretching

3 Components to Your Exercise Routine

You will be able to address each of the five components of fitness by incorporating something from each of these three categories of exercise into your overall plan. A well-rounded fitness routine includes something from each of three main categories of exercise, but you have many choices in each of these categories. You have choices in how balanced you spread out your efforts in these three areas, as well as choices in activity, intensity, and complexity. Here's a brief overview. Next, I've devoted an entire chapter to each area.

1. Aerobic Exercise

Description

Aerobic exercise is any activity that, through using many large muscle groups, increases your breathing and heart rate for an extended period of time (traditionally twenty minutes or more). The key phrase is "extended period of time," meaning that the activity or intensity that *you* can sustain for twenty minutes might not be the same as what your neighbor can sustain for twenty minutes. The literal translation of the word "aerobic" means "with oxygen," therefore, it reflects the ability of your body to continually deliver the oxygen necessary to do the work as you go along. If the workload is too hard (such as an all-out sprint down the street), you'll soon need to stop, put your hands on your knees and "suck wind" — panting to catch your breath. That would be "anaerobic" or without oxygen. You didn't have enough oxygen to continue so you had to stop and breathe in extra oxygen to make up for what you lost.

Examples

Examples of aerobic exercise include brisk walking, jogging, aerobics classes, stair-climber machines, elliptical trainer machines, cross-country ski machines, swimming, and cycling. Remember that whether each of these activities is truly aerobic for you depends on your fitness level. (You might be able to sustain brisk walking, but jogging might be too intense for it to be considered aerobic for you. Or maybe you can sustain a slow jog, but not a fast jog.)

Benefits

The benefits of aerobic exercise are far-reaching, making it a favorite of any fitness enthusiast. As for how aerobic exercise impacts the components of fitness, it improves your cardiovascular endurance, body composition, and muscular endurance. The cardiovascular and body composition benefits are delivered on an overall basis, while the muscular endurance benefits are based on the muscles that are primarily used for the activity. The benefits don't stop with those three major components of fitness. The list goes on and on! As aerobic exercise improves your heart health, it also decreases your risk of heart disease, diabetes, certain cancers, and a host of other diseases and ailments. And because you burn so many calories per minute of aerobic exercise, it helps with weight loss and/or weight maintenance. If the activity is weight bearing (meaning that you're standing up during it), it improves bone density, which decreases your risk of osteoporosis. Quite a list, huh?

2. Resistance Training

Description

Resistance training targets each muscle group, one by one, with the intention of fatiguing that muscle by applying some kind of weight against it when the muscle contracts. The resistance has to be challenging in order to gain significant benefits — you can't just go through the motions.

Examples

Examples of resistance training include weight-training exercises using free weights and dumbbells, single station and multi-station weight-training exercise machines such as Universal or Nautilus machines, elastic tubing, calisthenics and body weight exercises like push-ups and crunches, and "body sculpting" type group exercise classes.

Benefits

Resistance training increases muscular strength, muscular endurance, and improves body composition. You'll get stronger, firmer muscles, with the specific results of strength vs. endurance being dependent upon how heavy the resistance is for you and how much you do. Recall that if you use a higher weight with fewer repetitions you are building more strength. If you are using a comparatively lighter weight and perform more repetitions, you will build primarily endurance. Either way, the increase in muscle that you gain from resistance training increases your metabolic rate to allow you to burn more calories at rest, during exercise, and all throughout the day.

3. Stretching

Description

Stretching exercises also need to target each specific muscle group. By gently moving a muscle until it is fully extended, you will increase the flexibility of those muscle fibers. Stretches are best performed slowly and gently to the point of mild tension and then held in that position.

Examples

There are specific positions that stretch each major muscle group. An example would be lying on the floor on your back and holding your knees into your chest. This position stretches your lower back muscles. Yoga and Pilates can also improve flexibility.

Benefits

The benefits of stretching exercises are improved flexibility of the muscle that is targeted. You can increase your range of motion for that muscle which usually translates to greater ease of movement and reduced risk of injury. Stretching can also provide relief for stress-induced muscle tension and help rehabilitate any number of overuse injuries such as tendonitis or a strained muscle.

Next Steps

It's time to take a closer look at each of the three categories of exercise to start thinking about how to best fit things together for your solution.

The 5 Components of Fitness:

- ❒ Cardiovascular Endurance / Aerobic Fitness
- ❒ Muscular Strength
- ❒ Muscular Endurance
- ❒ Flexibility
- ❒ Body Composition

The 3 Components to Your Exercise Routine:

- ❒ Aerobic Exercise
- ❒ Resistance Training
- ❒ Stretching

How They Match Up:

- ❒ Aerobic Exercise = cardio endurance, muscular endurance, and body composition
- ❒ Resistance Training = muscular strength, muscular endurance, and body composition
- ❒ Stretching = flexibility

Chapter 6

Aerobic Exercise

Aerobic exercise can be the simplest part of your exercise routine. Or, if you become a real fitness enthusiast, there are dozens of ways to manipulate the different components to alleviate boredom, improve your results, or customize your efforts. We'll take a close look at the traditional guidelines for aerobic exercise, but remember that when we get to the Busy Mom Exercise Levels section, you will be able to choose how simple vs. complex, minimalist vs. comprehensive that you want to get with your program. It's usually best to start simple and see where your interest takes you in the future.

Opportunities for aerobic exercise are all around us. They can be solo activities, group activities, or family activities. Walking, jogging, and running all fit the bill for different people. There's bike riding with the kids, and all kinds of stationary equipment at home or at the gym — stationary bicycles, elliptical trainers, stair climber machines, cross country ski machines, and treadmills. How about a class — step aerobics or cardio kickboxing anyone? How about swimming? Remember, finding an activity you enjoy should be at the top of your decision-making list.

We've already touched on the major benefits of aerobic exercise — that it fabulously improves your cardiovascular endurance, your muscular endurance, and body composition.

I'd love to share some additional details and interesting facts about all you have to gain from aerobic exercise, as there are a host of other benefits! Remember, being able to appreciate and visualize what's happening in your body might be just enough of an extra push to get you jumping on the bandwagon.

Aerobic exercise is a great way to burn calories and thereby reduce fat, regardless of where it is on your body (and remember, you can't pick where you want it to come off of anyway). You may be burning anywhere from six to twelve calories per minute while exercising (as opposed to approximately one calorie per minute at rest). Because of this, aerobic exercise is your best chance to burn a large number of calories in a short amount of time, increasing the total number of calories you burn in a day. In addition, the extra calorie burning doesn't stop with the workout itself. Depending upon your intensity, your body may continue to burn calories at a higher rate for several hours after each aerobic workout. Therefore, the more often you engage in aerobic exercise, the more benefits you'll see. In fact, when you regularly engage in aerobic exercise, your body makes changes that allow you to burn more calories *all day long.* Do you remember the term "mitochondria" from high school biology? I still remember the exact definition from when I was in high school — a mitochondria is the "powerhouse of the cell" — the calorie burning, energy creating force within the cells of your body. Regular aerobic exercise causes your body *to increase the size and number of mitochondria* in your muscle cells. Pretty cool adaptation, huh? More mitochondria equals increased metabolic activity at rest as well as during activity. You will burn more calories all throughout the day because your muscle cells will be in a more constant state of vibration — like Mexican jumping beans!

Aerobic exercise not only burns a large number of calories during your workout, it also increases your calorie-burning capacity all day long!

Your Fat-Releasing Friend

So you want to *"burn fat,"* huh? There's no doubt that most of us have plenty of fat to burn. The problem is that the fat is in our fat cells, and we've got to get it out of the fat cells and transported to the muscle cells to do the burning. Do you have fat that is trapped in your fat cells? Have you ever wondered how and why fat is released from your fat cells? You've probably guessed that it involves aerobic exercise! Hold onto your hat for a little more scientific terminology, based on a lively presentation by my Canadian colleague, Andrè Noël Potvin.

There's an enzyme in your body called hormone sensitive lipase (but you can call it HSL). HSL is your friend and HSL's very important job is to sit along the border of your fat cells and release fat into the bloodstream to be used for energy. As long as HSL keeps dumping fat into the bloodstream, you can continue using it for fuel.

Guess what two things increase HSL? Drum roll, please . . . 1) Long term (meaning years) of consistent aerobic exercise and 2) increased activity throughout the day on a regular basis. If you've got a lifetime of exercise behind you, your HSL level will stay nice and high, even if you take a break for sickness or vacation. Your long history together has trained your HSL friends that you'll need them again soon, even when you take a break. If you're within the first few years of a new exercise habit, you will acquire more HSL friends, but they don't yet get the message that they are needed for life. When you take a week or two off from exercise, some of them will disappear, assuming that you no longer need them.

HSL

What it does:
Releases fat to be used as energy

Increased by:
1) Long-term aerobic exercise
2) Increased activity throughout the day.

Need an illustration of this concept? Let's talk marathon runners. You may think that marathon runners are among the most fit people on the planet. For the most part, they are, but all marathon runners are not created equal. Let's take an elite marathon runner. She's been training for a decade and may have as many as 30,000 HSLs! She can run for hours at a 5-minute mile pace (a crazy-fast pace for most people for even one block), but since she's got so *many* HSL friends, she's able to access a ton of fat to get the job done. That's also the reason why she can sustain such a fast pace for the entire marathon. Remember fat usage and on-going oxygen usage go hand in hand. Normal mortals can barely do the 100-yard dash at that speed and would need to stop and suck some serious wind at the end — replacing all the oxygen they didn't have to do the job. Also, since our elite marathoner uses so much fat, she hasn't needed to dip into her glucose stores as much. Want to know one organ that relies solely on glucose and can't use fat as fuel? The brain. So, since her muscles didn't have to steal her brain's glucose supply, our elite marathon runner finishes the marathon feeling great and celebrating with her friends.

As your body gets more efficient at using fat for fuel, it gets better at conserving glucose for when you really need it.

You'll be able to work out harder and still feel great!

Now let's take the novice marathon runner who has been training for only a year. Her HSL might only be 500 (as compared to 30,000!). She may still very well finish the marathon, but in addition to using fat as fuel, she'll use up every drop of glucose in her system. Chances are, with her muscles fighting for all the available glucose in her system, her brain (which can only function properly with glucose) has gotten shortchanged. As she crosses the finish line, she's stumbling, a little disoriented, and proud as can be but making very little sense!

Is this story supposed to make you feel badly? For Pete's sake, if a year of marathon training isn't enough to get you fit, why bother? Smile and take a breath. The scientific message is that as your body gets more efficient at using fat for fuel, it gets better at conserving glucose for when you really need it. You'll be able to work out harder and still feel great. Don't forget, also, the other way you can increase your HSL friends – consistent daily activity throughout the day. When you ask your body to move throughout the day, you're asking it over and over to mobilize fat and your body will get the message that it needs to get more efficient at releasing fat to get the job done. The motivational message is once again that fitness is a lifelong activity. Your body will continue to make adaptations based on years of living your life this way. Remember there is no finish line. You'll reap benefits for years and years!

Other Amazing Adaptations

An increased amount of fat circulating in the bloodstream increases the likelihood that your muscle cells will slurp it up and use it for fuel, but that's not guaranteed. We also need adaptations on the other end – the muscle cells' ability to absorb the fat out of the bloodstream. Aerobic exercise improves the ability of your muscles to absorb both fat and glucose out of the bloodstream. Another adaptation to regular aerobic exercise is the creation of additional capillaries (tiny blood vessels) surrounding the muscles in order to maximize the delivery of oxygen. It's like a highway construction crew has been called in to pave some new roads because they know there's going to be a lot of traffic coming through! The muscle cells themselves increase in size, endurance and tone through such repeated use and thus require more nutrients and calories to burn. What a great job you've done for yourself!

Aerobic exercise improves the ability of your muscles to absorb both fat and glucose from the bloodstream.

How Often, How Hard, and How Long?

Okay, we're done with the science for now. I'll bet you feel ready to jump right in! Let's get to the details that make a certain type of exercise count as an aerobic activity. Remember that in order to be considered aerobic, an exercise needs to use large muscle groups and elevate your heart rate for an extended period of time. The traditional criteria that need to be met in order to gain the benefits of aerobic exercise have been outlined by the American College of Sports Medicine (www.acsm.org, a great resource, by the way). They fall into the following categories:

Criteria to Gain the Benefits of Aerobic Exercise:

1. Frequency:

   typically 3–5 times per week

2. Intensity:

   typically within your
   "target heart rate zone"

3. Duration:

   typically 20–60 minutes

Let's take a look at each criterion in more detail . . .

"How often?" — Frequency

The traditional guidelines recommend that you do some form of aerobic exercise at least three times per week. The reasoning is that three times in a week gives your body a frequent enough stimulus to force it to adapt and compensate. The fitness principles of *overload* and *overcompensation* should make sense. If you place a demand on your body that it is not used to, your body will make the necessary adaptations to be able to rise to the occasion in the future. The muscle adaptation system (I like to call it the muscle memory system) really kicks in with a frequency of three times per week. If you exercise less than three times per week, your body "forgets" what happened by the time you do it again. Your body may be thinking, "Why overcompensate when I'm not asked to work this hard very often?"

You may be wondering, *"What about doing aerobic exercise more than three times per week?"* It is common for an aerobics enthusiast to do some kind of aerobic exercise as little as three times per week, up to five or even seven days per week. Seven days per week is a little extreme — one day of rest is always a good idea, especially for your joints. There is a general principle of diminishing returns, however, and the risk of something called "over-training." If you are doing more and more exercise and seeing less results, your body may be telling

This is a good time to check in with an all-or-none mindset test. Is your brain seeing all the possibilities and remembering that *any* amount of aerobic exercise is a great thing?

you it needs a break. However, some people really enjoy their exercise time and want to do it almost every day. If they are careful to sprinkle in at least several days a week with low intensity, easy-on-the-joints activities (like walking), they may be able to exercise seven days a week without a problem. If you're a seven-days-a-week kind of exerciser, you should definitely take a day off every now and then and make sure you mix up your modes of exercise so that you are not always stressing the same muscles and joints the same ways every time. Four or five days a week is more common for the well initiated. Obviously, the more days per week you are exercising, the more calories you will burn and the higher your cardiovascular conditioning. Busy moms who are mostly concerned with general conditioning are going to get great benefits with just three days per week. Busy moms who are trying to lose weight will probably find that they need more days per week (five is a good goal) in order to really impact weight loss.

"How hard?" — Intensity

There are many ways to measure or estimate the appropriate intensity for aerobic exercise. Remember that the goal for aerobic exercise is to work at an intensity that you can sustain for twenty minutes or more. (Some individuals, especially those who are very overweight, might start with even less than twenty minutes and that's okay!) There are several factors that determine whether you will want to measure your intensity more accurately or use a less-exact method of estimation. Let's look at the different methods you have to choose from, in order of simplest to most complex.

1. The "Talk Test"

You should feel like you can talk while you are exercising but you should prefer not to talk very much! If you feel like you can't talk at all, your intensity is probably too high. If you feel like you could gab at length while exercising, your intensity is probably not high enough!

2. **"Rate of Perceived Exertion" (RPE)**

There is a scale that rates your subjective perception of how hard you are exercising. Originally designed by Dr. Gunnar Borg, it is sometimes called the "Borg Scale." In most cases, your perception is closely linked to how fast your heart is beating (which is one of the hallmarks for determining exercise intensity). General advice for beginner fitness enthusiasts is that the exercise should feel "somewhat hard." For more advance exercisers, "hard" is okay, too. If you're RPE is between 13–15, or even 12–16 on the scale below, you are most likely in your aerobic zone. Anything else on the scale means your heart is probably beating too fast or too slow for an aerobic workout.

Borg-RPE-Scale:®

6	**No exertion at all**
7	
	Extremely light
8	
9	**Very light**
10	
11	**Light**
12	
13	**Somewhat hard**
14	
15	**Hard (heavy)**
16	
17	**Very Hard**
18	
19	**Extremely hard**
20	**Maximal exertion**

3. Target Heart Rate

Target heart rate zone training is the method of measuring intensity that is commonly used in health clubs and other formal exercise settings. First you find out what your "target heart rate zone" is and then you measure your heart rate during aerobic exercise to see if it is within that range. If your heart rate is higher than the top end of your target heart rate zone, you should exercise a little *less* vigorously. If your heart rate is lower than the bottom end of your zone, you should exercise a little *more* vigorously!

How to Find Your Target Heart Rate Zone

Target heart rate is based upon you having a maximum speed with which your heart can beat. This is called your maximum heart rate. We measure heart rate in *beats per minute* (bpm). Individuals vary, but the generally accepted method of estimating your maximum heart rate in beats per minute is the formula "220 minus your age." It is around this number that we reach absolute exhaustion. We do not exercise at our maximum heart rates! Rather, effective aerobic exercise involves doing the amount of work that makes our heart beat between 60–85% of our maximum heart rate. This range is called your "Target Heart Rate Zone." It's important to remember that this is a range, and that anything within that range is acceptable, unless you are doing advanced heart rate training.

During exercise, it's not practical to stop exercising for a whole minute to count your heart rate, so it is common practice to only count for 10 seconds and multiply by 6 to convert to beats per minute. The chart that follows has already done this for you. Simply refer to it and note your "zone" for the 10-second count. It should be a fairly easy range of numbers to remember once you get used to it.

When you exercise, take your heart rate to check whether or not you are in your target heart rate zone. Or better yet, wear a heart rate monitor that will continuously tell you what your heart rate is during your workout. If necessary, adjust how hard you are working. If your heart rate is below the zone, work a little harder; if your heart rate is above the zone, ease up a little. If you are somewhere in the middle, you're right where you should be!

How to Measure Your Heart Rate

Keeping your index finger and middle finger tightly together, place the pads (not the tips) of those fingers firmly on the inside of the opposite wrist, just below the base of the thumb. You may need to move your fingers around a bit to find the right spot, but be patient. Sooner or later, you should feel a pulsating sensation. Once you find it, count how many beats you feel in 10 seconds.

Target Heart Rate Zone

(Age)	*(Beats per minute)*	*(10-second count)*
20	**120–170**	**20–28**
25	**117–165**	**19–28**
30	**114–161**	**19–27**
35	**111–157**	**18–26**
40	**108–153**	**18–25**
45	**105–143**	**17–24**
50	**102–144**	**17–24**
55	**99–140**	**16–23**
60	**96–136**	**16–22**
65	**93–132**	**15–22**
70	**90–128**	**15–21**
75	**87–123**	**14–20**

A Customized Heart Rate Zone

One of the newest, most exciting technologies in fitness is the increased accessibility and affordability of metabolic testing equipment. I currently use this technology for my own clients. Recent studies suggest that the typical formula for estimating maximum heart rate is not accurate for some individuals, although until recently, that was all that was available. Even now, given no other choice, it should be used and you will still benefit. However, if you are looking for a more customized approach, check out this new technology. With a simple fitness test that measures your heart rate, oxygen consumption, and carbon dioxide production at the same time, it is possible to determine exactly the heart rate zone that is most effective for you for both fitness improvement and fat burning! You can find out more at my website, www.testyourmetabolism.com or at the website for New Leaf Health and Fitness, who developed the technology that I use: www.newleaffitness.com. It's great stuff! Sometimes a small adjustment in your target heart rate zone can make a huge difference in your results.

"How long?" – Duration

How long does your aerobic workout need to be? We've already established that 20 minutes is the traditional minimal recommendation for cardiovascular benefits. *However*, research now shows that there is much to be gained from shorter amounts of exercise, especially as compared to doing nothing! We'll get more into this later, but let's deal with the 20-60 minute time frame for now. The 20-minute recommendation is based primarily on improving cardiovascular fitness and heart health. If you are interested in losing weight, however, you will probably find that 20 minutes isn't quite enough. The more committed and enthusiastic types, and those who want to lose weight, often spend 30, 40, or even 60 minutes doing their aerobic workout. It is definitely the kind of thing that you need to build up. Also, it should make sense that the duration and the intensity are closely linked. On days that you decide to have a long workout, you will probably lower your intensity a bit to be able to continue for that long. Conversely, on days that are shorter, you may find that you can push yourself a little . . . or not! Either way is fine. In general, it is a great idea to vary the duration of your aerobic workouts. Maybe you'll decide to do several 20-minute workouts during the week and use the weekend to try to get in a longer one. It's important not to get caught up with "I should go longer" on any particular day or just in general. The longer workouts are only suitable if you enjoy them and they fit your schedule. Any amount of time is fabulous!

Be Careful What the Machines Tell You

Have you ever noticed that many of the treadmills, elliptical machines, and other types of aerobic equipment supposedly tell you how many calories you've burned during your workout? I wouldn't be too quick to believe those numbers. If the machine doesn't ask you to input your body weight, the calculation will have no validity at all. But, even with your body weight, the number may not be accurate for you, depending on your unique metabolism. It may be fun to watch the "calories burned" reading increase as you work out, just don't place much stock in the exact number.

Dispelling A Few Myths

"You don't burn fat until after 20 minutes."

Some people have heard you're not burning fat until after 20 minutes of aerobic exercise and that if you stop before 20 minutes, "you're not doing anything." This is simply not the case. For exercise sessions lasting less than one hour, intensity is the primary factor that determines the ratio of fat to glucose used, not time. Blood glucose and glucose already stored in your muscles get things started off, but fat usage increases right away. During aerobic exercise, you are always burning a combination of fat and glucose simultaneously. Recall that aerobic means "with oxygen" and metabolism that uses a continual oxygen supply allows fat to be released from your fat cells for energy. The fat-to-glucose ratio does gradually change the longer you exercise. As you deplete your muscle glycogen and blood sugar, fat supplies a higher percentage of the fuel, but you'd have to be exercising for close to two hours before it made a significant difference. Therefore, only athletes who train for marathons or triathlons need be concerned with such things.

"Low intensity burns more fat."

The notion of the "fat burner" class used to be very popular in health clubs. Women would do really low intensity exercise on purpose, thinking that they were burning more fat than if they were working harder. *Does lower intensity aerobic exercise burn more fat?* And do you need to use more fat as the fuel for a particular workout in order to lose more fat? While it is true that very low intensity exercise burns a higher percentage of fat as fuel, the total calories burned are lower, and thus, usually the fat calories are lower also. Slightly higher intensity aerobic exercise burns more total calories, which usually translates to more total fat. When the intensity is too intense (beyond your aerobic zone), there's no time for the oxygen-fat metabolism pathway. Fat usage plummets at this point, termed "anaerobic threshold." You'd know if you were in this glucose-only anaerobic zone because you wouldn't be able to hold out for long, and you'd need to breathe hard at the end to replace the oxygen you depleted. Metabolic exercise testing, which I mentioned in the previous section, is the only way to quantify how many total calories and fat calories per minute your body burns for a given heart rate. In my experience performing metabolic exercise tests, I have seen quite a variety of responses from person to person. And, in fact, I have tested many individuals whose fat usage plummeted at a lower intensity than expected. Expect to see much more in the area of metabolic fitness training in the coming years. Wouldn't it be great if such testing became commonplace so that each person could know exactly what heart rate corresponded to the most effective calorie and fat burning zone for them?

Scientific testing aside, I think the best way to handle intensity is to gauge the middle ground. Stay within your aerobic range and work as hard as you can for as long as you can within the 20–60 minute window that feels right for you. You will burn the same number of calories whether you walk or jog a given distance. The difference is how long it takes. A 45-minute walk vs. a 30-minutes jog will probably cover the same distance. Which can you handle? Which do you want to handle? What are you in the mood for? How much time do you have? How much joint stress can you withstand? You see, there are more questions than answers! And not all answers are black and white. Sometimes it's best not to overanalyze all the particulars. Do what feels right within the recommended parameters and vary it often. Most importantly, recognize that it's all good and get back to the notion of movement for pleasure!

Variation

It is a good idea to vary the kind of aerobic exercise that you do. For instance, I wouldn't recommend that you *always* do step aerobics or *only* jog. It is good to vary the method of exercise so that you are not stressing the same muscles and joints the same way with each workout. This will help prevent overuse injuries. It is especially unwise to do high impact exercises, such as running, *all the time,* as this really puts a lot of stress on your joints. Also, from a fitness improvement standpoint, you want to keep your body guessing. If you always do the same workout the same way, your body gets very efficient at it and you won't reap as many benefits as if you switched things around every now and then.

Interval Training: An Advanced Aerobic Training Method

Getting committed and getting started are both great things! But, what if you are already a regular aerobic exerciser? You may be looking for a little something to increase your benefit and decrease boredom. **Interval training** may be just the thing for you. It may sound complicated, but it really doesn't have to be. When you do interval training, you interject high intensity bursts occasionally throughout your normal aerobic exercise intensity. The high intensity intervals can be as short as 30 seconds, or as long as 3 minutes. Try sprinkling in just one or two of these bursts into your normal workout. If you like it, add even more intervals. While on your normal walk, pick a landmark about 50 yards ahead and walk as fast as possible until you get there, then slow down to your normal pace for the next 5 minutes and try it again. An even more challenging way to do intervals is to:

- maintain the higher intensity for 3–5 minutes and then . . .
- come back down to your lower intensity level for only one minute before . . .
- going back up to the high intensity level.

Now that's a workout!

Sometimes a shock to your system is just what the doctor ordered. In this way, you teach your body to tolerate the higher levels of work, but in small bits. Before you know it, you are able to elevate the overall intensity of your workout, thus burning more calories and more fat per minute the entire time.

Making Decisions and Putting Together Your Routine

For now, there's been a lot to absorb about how aerobic exercise works and what it can do for you. In a few more chapters, we'll get to the part where you'll use all this knowledge to put together the solution that works for you and your needs.

Chapter 7

Resistance Training

Throughout this book, I'll use the terms resistance training, weight training, and strength training interchangeably. Whatever you call it, and whether you're using free weights, machines, elastic tubing, or your own body weight, when you use muscular force *against a resistance,* it forces your muscles to respond and adapt. I like to call resistance training the *Secret Weapon* for women! Almost any kind of exercise will have a positive impact on your muscles, but resistance training is *the most powerful way* to do so. And, as a woman and busy mom, you have much to gain from building those muscles. In a nutshell, as related to the components of fitness, resistance training increases muscular strength, muscular endurance, and improves your body composition. Read on for motivating details about these primary benefits, as well as many more bonuses! Young or old, thin or heavy — weight training equals increased metabolism, a firmer looking body, better blood sugar regulation, and more stable joints. You can't afford *not* to do some form of resistance training!

If it's so great, why do many women shy away from resistance training? Check out the reasons listed on the following page. Do you see yourself in any of these scenarios?

Blocks to Resistance Training:

- Many women stick with what they know — which is usually limited to aerobic exercise.
- Some women think that if their primary objective is losing weight, they should just pile on more aerobic exercise. They figure they'll start weight training *after* they lose weight.
- Some are put off by misconceptions that lifting weights is a "guy's thing."
- Some are worried that they'll build unsightly bulky muscles.
- Some are intimidated by the machines and don't want to look silly.

Have No Fear!

Whatever your hesitation, by the end of this chapter, your fears will be put at ease. In fact, let's start by dispelling some of the more common weight training myths.

Don't Fall Prey to These Myths

"If I stop exercising, the muscle will turn to fat."

Muscle is muscle and fat is fat. They are completely different entities. Muscle never turns to fat and vice versa. That being said, here's the real scoop: When you begin a weight-training program, your muscles will get firmer and stronger, (and maybe *slightly* bigger, but not all that much to the naked eye) and your metabolism increases. When you stop your weight-training program, the muscle gets weaker, softer, and smaller. Your metabolism slows down, which causes your body to store more fat. The muscle has decreased and the fat has increased.

"Weight training will give me big, bulky muscles."

There are two things necessary to build big, bulky muscle: a lot of testosterone and an extremely demanding weight-training routine. Most women have neither. While women do have some testosterone in their bodies, they have far less of this hormone than men, which is why men can build muscle more easily. What about those really muscular women and female bodybuilders? Rest assured, their weight-training program looks nothing like the weight-training program of the typical woman who'd like to improve her health and appearance. Your weight-training routine would probably consist of three times per week, 10-40 minutes, at a moderate intensity. Female bodybuilders, because they are trying to build large muscles on purpose, have routines that last several hours per day, every day, lifting very heavy weights in a pretty grueling fashion! On top of that, some of them even take steroids – an artificial form of testosterone, which helps them build more muscle than they could on their own.

"If I want to lose fat from my stomach, I should do lots of abdominal work."

Hopefully, the myth of spot reduction is dying as more and more women learn the truth about exercise and how it works. I've said this before – you cannot pick where you want to lose fat, period. (Well, with the exception of liposuction!) Remember that fat loss happens on an overall basis and based on your genetics. It often happens from top to bottom – meaning the first thing you'll hear when you lose a little weight is "Your face looks thinner." *(Thanks, Mom.)* Next, your collarbones may become a little more prominent, and then the waistband of your jeans gets looser. Last, last, last, for many women is the hip and thigh area! For other women, the last to go will be the "pooch" on your stomach area. As frustrating as this is, your body will decide where it wants to release the fat, which is rarely where you'd like it come from! After all, it wouldn't be your "problem area" if your body was particularly anxious to shed fat from that area, now would it? Supermodels aside, we all have a body type, whether you are thin or heavy. The common terms for these two types are apple – and pear-shaped. Apples, even when they are at their ideal weight, may still be frustrated with their stomach. Pears at their ideal weight, will most likely still carry some in the "saddlebag" area. I still remember an old friend passing along her boyfriend's comment when she expressed frustration about her outer thigh area. He remarked quite nonchalantly, "It's not going anywhere so you might as well learn to love it!" Imagine *loving* your trouble spot? Not just putting up with it or accepting it, but *loving* it. Isn't that a great notion?

Getting back to the impact of weight training . . . it can indeed, help the look of your problem area even if it doesn't help you lose fat from the area. When there is a strong, firm muscle beneath the fat, the overall appearance of that body part will be improved. Just remember that those exercises aren't working on the fat that lies on top of the muscles in that area. Common problem areas include the back of the arm, the stomach area, and the thighs. Doing triceps exercises, crunches, and squats, for example, will firm up the muscles in those body areas, but will not decrease the layer of fat lying on top of those muscles.

The Top Five Benefits of Resistance Training

Now that we've covered some things that resistance training doesn't do, let's get to what it does do. You can expect the following fabulous benefits when you embark on a weight-training program:

Increased Round-the-Clock Metabolism

When you think of burning calories, do you automatically think of exercise? Think again! The truth is that even when you are just sitting around, doing nothing, your body is burning calories. And in fact, your resting metabolic rate (the number of calories your body burns twenty-four hours a day, even at rest) typically contributes 60–75% of the total number of calories you burn in a day! One estimate of your calorie burn rate at rest is approximately one calorie per minute, or 60 calories per hour. Muscle is one of the most important factors that determine whether *you* burn slightly more or less than the one calorie per minute estimate, making weight training possibly the single best investment you can make in increasing your resting metabolic rate. And when you impact your resting metabolic rate, you impact total calories in a big way. If your metabolism is like a fire, then the muscle cell is a *furnace*. Your muscle cell is "the" *calorie-burning machine* in your body. Weight training increases the size and efficiency of your muscle cells giving you a larger and stronger furnace. Therefore, the more muscle you have, the more calories you burn all throughout the day — at rest, while going about the business of your day, and during exercise. Do you burn many calories during your weight-training workout itself? Well, not really . . . especially when compared to aerobic exercise for the same amount of time. The important thing to keep in mind is that the benefits of weight training are not measured in a single workout. Rather, weight training is an investment in total calories that you burn *the other twenty-three hours of the day.* Important stuff! All of this information might explain why men usually have an advantage when it comes to metabolism. We've all heard the complaint; *"**He** can eat anything without gaining weight!"* Well, it's a valid gripe! Pound for pound, when comparing a man and a woman of the same weight, the man will have substantially more

The more muscle you have, the more calories you burn, all day long.

muscle on his body every time, hands down. This doesn't give women an easy out, though. It does give women all the more reason to do what they can to increase their muscle mass! Because many women are starting with smaller muscles, they sometimes see the *greatest* gains when they begin a strength-training program! If you are not doing some form of weight training, you are missing a valuable opportunity to impact your metabolism.

A Firmer-looking Body

Muscle provides the shape and contour of our body. Aerobic exercise is wonderful and will always be wonderful. But, if you are doing *only* aerobic exercise, you are missing the opportunity to change the *shape* of your body. When you lose weight through diet and aerobic exercise alone, you may lose weight, but you may also end up with simply a smaller version of your current body shape. Let's say you consider yourself pear-shaped. I doubt your goal is to become a smaller pear. Through weight training, you will be able to shape and sculpt the muscles that provide the contours of your body.

You may be wondering about that ever-present layer of fat on top of the muscles. Yes, it is true that you won't quite see the contours (i.e. the "cut" muscles) if you have a thick layer of fat on top. But, you *will* still see a difference. Every body part will look firmer with a strong muscle as its foundation. Of course you can still take measures to reduce the layer of fat on top of the muscle at the same time. What's the key there? Eating habits, aerobic exercise, and . . . weight training . . . again! As I already mentioned, weight training contributes to fat loss by increasing muscle, which increases calories burned all day.

A Stronger You

We need muscular strength a lot more than we think to get through our daily activities. "Use it or lose it" definitely applies. Whether you're holding a twenty-three-pound "baby" on your hip all day, or schlepping groceries into the house, strong muscles will serve you well and stave off aches and pains. Muscles that are used to working hard respond to difficulties by rebuilding even stronger for next time. I'm sure you can think of endless ways to put your newfound strength and energy to good use — getting more things done each day, tiring those kids out (instead of the other way around), and certainly leaping small buildings with a single bound!

Help with Blood Sugar Regulation

Working muscles need fuel, and when muscles spend a lot of time working, they get really good at absorbing fuel. Muscle cells need to extract energy (glucose) from the bloodstream and they need to be receptive to the hormone insulin to do so. An inactive muscle may have a hard time letting insulin do its job of escorting glucose to the muscle cells. The glucose is there, it's in the bloodstream . . . but it can't get into the muscle where it needs to be. So, the body compensates by dumping even more insulin into the bloodstream trying to get the muscles to listen. Hmmm. Does increased insulin and increased blood sugar floating aimlessly around the bloodstream sound familiar? (You guessed right if you're thinking about a breeding ground for diabetes.) To put icing on the cake, there is one location that will eagerly accept all that homeless blood sugar and loves high insulin levels . . . your fat cells! So, strong muscles and regular exercise can change your body's chemistry and hormones, and help your muscle cells slurp up blood sugar before the fat cells can get to it. Any takers?

Increased Joint Stability

When you think of the location of a muscle (any muscle), you probably think about what body part that particular muscle covers. You know, biceps are on front of the upper arm, quadriceps are on the front of your thigh, etc. Am I right? I'd like to challenge you to picture something different in your mind. Think of which joint each muscle crosses. After all, the purpose of each muscle is to create movement. Every muscle in your body must cross one or more joints in order for this to happen. The biceps cross the elbow joint and the quadriceps cross the knee joint. The back and chest muscles both cross the shoulder joint and attach onto your upper arm. When the muscle is strong, it encases the joint in a more stable way and reduces the chance of injury to that joint. The strong muscle is better equipped to withstand an unexpected force placed on a joint when you stumble or have an accident. So, "having bad knees," for example, is not a good reason to avoid leg exercises . . . it's a reason to do them (carefully designed and supervised by a professional, of course)!

The Take-home Message

Have you figured out the message yet? *You need to be doing some form of resistance training exercise!* It doesn't have to be fancy. It doesn't have to be extensive. Whether you're young, old, injury-plagued, or just short on time, there is a strength-training routine that can work for you. Whether it's a fitness center routine, a 10-minute home program with a few sets of dumbbells and elastic tubing, or bicep curls with soup cans, there is so much to be gained. I'll show you lots of choices in the Busy Mom's Exercise Levels section.

How Resistance Training Works

Important Principle #1:

Overload, Rest, and Adaptation

The most important thing to keep in mind about resistance training is that muscles respond to overload. This means that in order for the muscle to get the message that it needs to adapt, the workload has got to be difficult. Just going through the motions is not going to cut it! When you work your muscles, you are, in fact, damaging them on a microscopic level. (Don't worry. This is a good thing!) The muscle responds by rebuilding stronger than ever. That is why you have probably heard that you shouldn't do weight training for the same muscle group two days in a row. The day of rest in between is just as important as the day of work. It is during that time that the muscle is rebuilding. If you work a muscle really hard day after day without a break, it doesn't have the opportunity to grow and repair itself.

Important Principle #2:
Progression

The amount of weight that overloads your muscles today will probably not be the weight that overloads your muscles six months from now if you're exercising consistently. As your muscles grow and your strength builds, you will need to challenge your new strength with heavier and heavier weights. Of course, there is a limit to your progression, especially based on how extensive your exercise routine is. (The woman doing one set per muscle group will plateau before the woman doing three sets per muscle group.) You will know when you get there, and then your job will shift to maintaining your fitness level. That being said, most women can benefit from at least attempting to lift heavier weights as the weeks and months go by. You may get stuck always doing your bicep curls with eight-pound dumbbells, for example because they feel "hard" enough when you do them. But when you finally give the ten-pound dumbbells a try, you might just find out that you can do them. Suddenly, you say to yourself, *"Those eights weren't that hard after all.* ***This*** *is hard!"* The very attempt to use heavier weights can re-set your idea of "what's hard." If they're too heavy, you can always go back, but at least you tried. You will know that they are too heavy if you can't perform the exercise with good form. Good form means being able to maintain proper body alignment and complete the entire range of motion without using momentum or needing to contort your body in any way to get through the movement. If you find yourself cheating (not going through the full range of motion) or compensating with another body part, you tried to move up too soon.

Important Principle #3:
Use It or Lose It

Muscles respond to the overload by growing and getting stronger. When the stimulus stops, the muscles gradually shrink and go back to the way they used to be. Unfortunately, you can't save up muscular fitness (or any other kind of fitness, for that matter). The benefits don't fade overnight if you stop, but over weeks or months, they will fade. In general, the benefits are only as good as the time you are engaging in that lifestyle. That's why it's important to keep it up and find a solution that you can maintain or adjust over time to combat boredom or life changes.

Important Principle #4:
Specificity

While the benefits of aerobic exercise include overall, non-specific fat loss, resistance training is a whole different story. Yes, there is the non-specific benefit of increased metabolism, but when it comes to increasing the strength and firmness of your muscles, the way to do so is by targeting each specific muscle group one at a time. There are certain exercises that target several related muscle groups together, but the fact remains that when you're well-informed, you go down your list of major muscle groups and make sure you hit each one.

Major Muscle Groups

For a comprehensive resistance training routine, you'll want to do one or more exercises for each of the following muscle groups. Remember, when we get to the Busy Mom's Exercise Levels, you may very well decide to only train a few of these muscle groups for now. You can tuck this information away for when you are ready for more!

Upper Body

- Shoulders
- Chest
- Back
- Biceps (front of the arm)
- Triceps (back of the arm)
- Abdominals (stomach area)

Lower Body

- Quadriceps (front of the thigh)
- Hamstrings (back of the thigh)
- Gluteus Maximus (rear end)
- Hips (note that your hip muscles are not on your outer thigh, they are above your hip joint)
- Inner Thigh

Good form means being able to maintain proper body alignment and complete the entire range of motion without using momentum or needing to contort your body in any way to get through the movement.

Muscles that Work Together

If you think about moving your body, very seldom does one muscle work alone. Most of the time, several muscle groups work together to cause movement, in exercise and in real life. Try to avoid thinking about what body part a muscle is positioned on, but rather, focus on what joint it crosses. For instance, getting up out of a chair requires your hip and knee joints to move, thus requiring both your quads and glutes to work together. Push-ups cause movement in your shoulder and elbow joints. Therefore, even though you think of push-ups as a chest exercise, they also work the triceps. What does this mean for your exercise routine? Quite simply, that you can make good use of combo exercises that work several muscle groups together. These are usually called "compound exercises." "Isolation exercises" that move only one joint at a time, and thus only work one muscle group at a time, can have a valuable place in your routine as well. We'll get to details on that in the Busy Mom's Advanced Exercise Level.

Tips for Sequencing Your Routine

In general, it is a good idea to work your large muscle groups before the smaller muscle groups that assist them. For instance, the triceps are involved in many chest exercises. If you work your triceps before your chest, you'll end up with arms that feel like spaghetti while you're trying to work your chest. The same rule applies for back and biceps. The biceps assist with your back exercises. Better to work the back first and then the biceps after that.

Weight Training Lingo and Important Info

You'll feel a whole lot more comfortable with your exercise routine if you know the lingo and the background information for setting up a sound program. Here are a few terms and principles that you must know and understand:

Repetitions

"Reps" means repetitions, the number of times you perform an exercise before stopping. Most women will do between 8-15 repetitions of an exercise. Perform each repetition carefully and purposefully — typically a little faster on the first part (contraction) and a bit slower when you are returning to your starting position. You can pace yourself by counting "one . . . two..." on the way up (or whenever the muscle is contracting) and "one . . . two . . . three . . . four..." on the way back down (or when the muscle is elongating again).

How Many Reps Should I Do?

It should make sense that the heavier the weight is, the less repetitions you can do, right? And conversely, the lighter the weight, the more repetitions you can do. The question is, which is better for your goals? Recall the fitness components of muscular strength and muscular endurance. I described muscular strength and muscular endurance as opposite ends along a continuum of resistance training. Traditional fitness guidelines recommend using heavier weights and fewer repetitions to work on the strength end of the continuum. Conversely, when you use lighter weights and do more repetitions, you are working on the endurance portion of the continuum. When you are right in the middle, you will get a little of both — something that fitness professionals like to call "general conditioning."

Twelve repetitions is the classic prescription for general conditioning, but it includes resistance training within the range of 8–15 repetitions. The newest research presented by the American College of Sports Medicine indicates *similar strength and endurance benefits when you reach momentary muscular fatigue anywhere within 8–15 repetitions.* This new research minimizes the applicability of the strength-endurance continuum within 8–15 repetitions. This is a slight departure from traditional guidelines that suggested an 8-repetition routine would result in more strength gains and a 15-repetition routine would result in more endurance gains. The most important factor is that you do indeed reach fatigue when you stop, at whatever number it happens to be within the 8–15 repetition range. The only difference within that range, according to the new research, has to do with bone density. The research shows superior improvements in bone density when you use heavier weights and reach fatigue within the lower (8–10) repetitions range as opposed to using lighter weights and reaching fatigue within the higher (14–15) repetition range — great for reducing your risk of osteoporosis.

Select the Weight that Causes You to Reach Fatigue with this Range of Repetitions

You don't just decide to perform 8–15 repetitions and end it there. The next important step is to select the weight that will cause you to reach fatigue within that range of repetitions. ***This is perhaps the most important piece of information about effective weight training!*** You don't just stop at 12 repetitions because that's your number to stop. "Going to fatigue," means that you *can't do any more.* Or more specifically, that you can't continue in *good form.*

For instance, if you find that you start throwing your body around, arching your back, or using momentum to complete an exercise, it's time to *stop*. You could do more harm than good at that point. For this reason, it is often helpful to have a full-body mirror available while you do you weight-training program. A mirror is a great tool to use for monitoring your form.

Moving Back and Forth between the Number of Reps You Perform Should Be Fluid

Figuring out what weight will get you to fatigue within 8–15 repetitions is a work in progress. Sometimes you overestimate or underestimate the weight that you can do for, say, 12 repetitions. If it's 11 repetitions that day, so be it. If it's 14, that's fine, too. You'll store that information away because it will help you decide when it's time to try the next weight up. For instance, when you first start lifting weights, eight-pound dumbbells may be what causes you to fatigue by 12 repetitions. Gradually, you

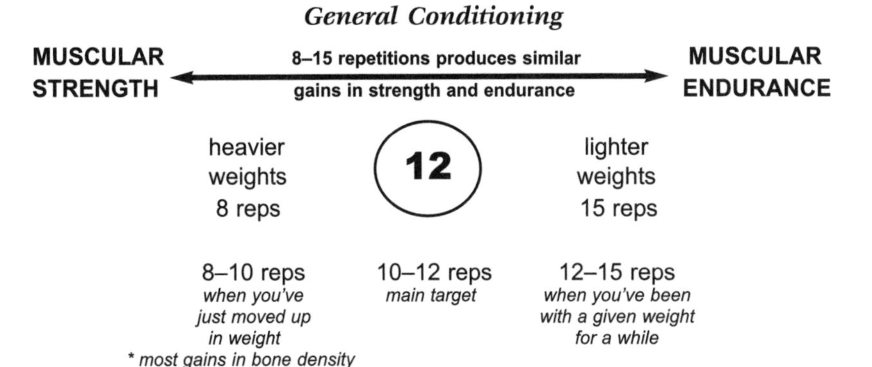

notice that 12 reps aren't that hard so you do 13, then 14 another day. Then you're back to 12 on a day that you're particularly tired. Once you get 14 or 15 reps consistently, it's time to try the 10-pound dumbbells. My rule of thumb is that if you can squeak out 8–10 reps when you go up in weight, it's a keeper. Then, as you stay with that weight, you'll probably work your way back up to 12 reps with the new weight. Then, over more weeks and months, you may start creeping back towards 15 reps again, so you're ready to up the weight *again!* If you always concentrate on "going to fatigue," you will always get maximum benefit out of the exercise. Many women make the mistake of staying with a given weight way too long. If they just tried the heavier weight, they would see that they could do it, and get more benefits because of it!

Sets

Once you complete your desired number of repetitions, you have completed one *set*. You may or may not do another set after resting that muscle group for a few minutes. For example, if you perform 12 repetitions of the bicep curl exercise, rest for a few minutes and then do 12 more, you have just completed 2 sets of bicep curls.

How Many Sets?

Most busy moms will do between 1–3 sets per muscle group. One set is the perfect place to start and is also where many people stay — it's quick and still beneficial. Two sets will give even more benefits, and three even more than that. There's no reason to feel locked into a particular program. Let it change and evolve as you have more and less time. If you know more than one exercise for each muscle group, you may want to mix it up even more, as long as you generally do the same number of sets for each muscle group. For instance, push-ups and dumbbell flies both work the chest muscles. If you typically do 2 sets per muscle group, you may decide to do 2 sets of push-ups, 2 sets of flies, or 1 set of each. The choice is yours and variety is a good thing. Your body responds well to surprises! I usually do my weight training routine on Monday, Wednesday, and Friday mornings. Some days I do 3 sets per muscle group, but if I oversleep or am otherwise in a hurry, I might just zip through 1 or 2 sets. Again, we'll get into the particulars in the Busy Mom's Exercise Levels.

How Often?

The general rule of thumb is to do your strength-training program three times per week — always with a day off in between. A more modest program may be twice a week and that is still beneficial. Remember that during your workout, you are microscopically shredding your muscle cells and that they need about forty-eight hours to repair themselves and grow stronger. That's why you generally skip a day between weight-training workouts. If the exercise is particularly light for you — not much resistance and you perform many, many repetitions (a good example is abdominal crunches), there's no problem doing that particular exercise every day or several days in a row.

How Long Will It Take?

We'll look at a variety of ways to set up your weight-training program in the Busy Mom's Exercise Levels section. The good news is that your entire routine could take as little as five to ten minutes or as long as an hour, depending on the number of sets you do per muscle group, which in turn is dependent upon your goals, time available, and enthusiasm. Remember, it's flexible and whether it's minimal or extensive, it's worthwhile!

A Summary of Resistance Training Principles:

- ✔ 2–3 times per week (always skip a day between)
- ✔ 1–3 sets per body part
- ✔ Repetitions: usually 8–15
- ✔ Select the weight based on what will fatigue you within that range of repetitions
- ✔ If you're not at fatigue by the end of your predetermined range of repetitions, keep going until you do reach fatigue and consider increasing the weight next time.

Chapter 8

Stretching

Stretching is often the overlooked and under-appreciated afterthought to many exercise routines. We hate to admit the reason why so many of us skimp on stretching — that it does nothing for our appearance! We realize that there are benefits to stretching, but unfortunately, none that we can see in the mirror. It does feel great, though, and has much to offer. In fact, stretching can be a great break when you've spent a little too much time in front of the computer, for example. You don't need to be in exercise clothes, and there is no sweating involved!

In Chapter 5, we covered the fact that stretching improves the flexibility of your muscles, which in turn can help you more comfortably reach and bend through a typical day, especially a day that involves other types of exercise.

Here are some tips to keep in mind about stretching:

- Remember that flexibility is specific to each muscle group. In order to "hit" each muscle group, you'll need to do a series of stretches, each targeting a specific muscle group.
- Flexibility is different in each person and is determined largely by genetics. Don't compare yourself to

others with regard to how far you can stretch. Concentrate on stretching correctly and to the point that your body can comfortably go.

- You should stretch slowly and gently to the point of mild tension (not pain) and then hold that position.
- How long should you hold each stretch? General guidelines recommend that you hold a stretch for 15–30 seconds for a mild stretch and up to 3 minutes if you are trying to improve a particular problem with a muscle.
- It is best not to bounce when you stretch. Think about what happens when you quickly stretch a rubber band. A quick, forceful stretch on the rubber does not result in a lengthened rubber band. Instead, it snaps back, doesn't it? This is a great analogy for your muscles. In addition to the contractile part of the muscle cells, there is a special part inside (called the muscle spindle) that acts like a motion detector. When the muscle spindles detect large, sudden movement, they send a message to the contractile part of the muscle to contract quickly, to protect itself from a muscle tear. This is the opposite of what you want since you are trying to stretch, not contract the muscle! So don't treat your muscles like a rubber band when you are trying to stretch. It is far better to gently sneak up on the muscle with a slow, gradual stretch.
- Stretching and warming up are not the same thing. Warming up involves doing some kind of light activity, (like walking or bicycling) for 3–5 minutes, which increases your circulation and body temperature. Stretching may also be done before your aerobic or resistance training workout, but only after the warm-up. Make sense? Once your circulation has increased and your muscles are warmer and filled with more blood, they are softer and more pliable, which makes them more receptive to stretching. This is why you may have heard that it's best not to stretch when your muscles are cold. When they are warm, they'll stretch like taffy and you'll get a much more effective stretch.

* Stretching before you work out, but after you warm up, is the best way to prepare for exercise. Stretching before exercise has been credited with decreasing the risk of injury during your workout. When you are stretching for flexibility gains, you are better off investing even more of your time *after* your workout when your muscles are really, really warm.
* How often should you stretch? Shoot for a minimum of 3 times per week in order to gain the benefits of regular stretching. If you enjoy it, stretching exercises can safely be done every day. In fact, if you are recovering from a chronic muscle injury, your doctor or physical therapist might suggest doing certain stretches 3–5 times per day, holding each stretch for several minutes.
* Refer to the photos and detailed descriptions in Appendix 2 for specific stretching exercises. Note that not every stretch will feel good for every body. Try out a new stretch gently for the first time to see if it's comfortable for you. Also, be sure to seek professional guidance from a fitness trainer if you are unsure about correct positioning or appropriateness of a particular stretch for you.

Stretching is Super

A regular stretching program will take you far in comfort and ease of movement during everyday life and as you age. Even though everyone's genetic potential for flexibility is different, the truth is that most of us are not reaching that potential. Years of disuse cause our muscles to shorten unnecessarily, creating an overall stiffness and a breeding ground for all sorts of aches and pains. Make sure you don't fall into the trap of using "I'm just not flexible," as an excuse not to stretch. A simple stretching routine several times per week can make a big difference for anyone. You can improve your flexibility and it is well worth it!

Time For A Stretch Break!

Any time you need to improve your mood, reduce fatigue, and ease stiff, achy muscles try this ***Quick Standing Stretch Break Sequence,*** *which stretches the upper back, shoulders, chest, neck, biceps, and triceps. Hold each position for 10-30 seconds before moving to the next step.*

1. Clasp your hands out in front of you with straight arms and press out, rounding your upper back.
2. Slowly raise your arms, hands still clasped together, above your head and press up.
3. Release your clasped hands, grab one wrist and tug upward. Change and grab the other wrist and tug upward.
4. Bring your arms down until your elbows are bent approximately 90 degrees (like field goal posts). Pull your arms back, squeezing your shoulder blades together.
5. Let your arms fall open, straightening your elbows with your palms facing up.
6. Press your arms down and out through the heel of your hands. Drop your head slowly to one side, then circle halfway around to the other side.
7. Lift one arm overhead, elbow bent, with your hand hanging down your back. With the fingertips of your opposite hand, pull back just above the elbow. Switch.

An Anytime Seated Back Relaxer

Sitting for an extended period of time can make your back feel tired. Here's a quick way to soothe and relax those lower back muscles.

1. Push away from your desk. Keep your feet planted on the floor wider than hip-width apart.
2. Lower your head, round your back, and slowly bend forward from the waist and hang down between your knees for 10 seconds. Gently uncurl, sit straight and relax.

Chapter 9

Putting It All Together

We've covered the basics in the areas of aerobic exercise, resistance training, and stretching. Now, it's time to take a quick look at a few other considerations that you should keep in mind when embarking on your new fitness lifestyle.

Health History

How's your health? It's important to check with your doctor before starting a vigorous exercise routine if you have a heart or lung problem, diabetes, bone or joint problem, or several of the risk factors for cardiovascular (heart) disease. Take a look at the list on the following pages of items that warrant a check-in with your doctor, based on guidelines by the American College of Sports Medicine (ACSM).

Warm-Up

It is important to ease your body into exercise. Whether you are about to do aerobic exercise, resistance training, or stretching, spending 3–5 minutes walking or doing some other form of light continuous movement is important to warm up.

(Remember that warming up literally means increasing your body temperature and that warming up and stretching are not the same thing.) In this way, you'll prepare your body for exercise by increasing circulation to your muscles that will soon need it.

Cool-Down

Cool-down applies specifically to aerobic exercise. It is recommended that you take 3–5 minutes at the end of your aerobic workout to walk slowly or simply do a lower intensity version of whatever activity you were doing. This will allow your heart rate to gradually lower back to a normal rate. Abruptly stopping your aerobic workout while you are at a high intensity can lead to dizziness or tingling legs as the blood tries desperately to climb back up to the brain against gravity without the help of your muscles continuing to contract. For people who are at a high risk for heart disease, the absence of a cool-down period can result in irregular heartbeats or other cardiac rhythm irregularities. Don't forget to cool down!

You should check with your doctor prior to beginning an exercise routine if:

- ❍ You are over 55 years of age (for men it's over 45 years of age).
- ❍ You have two or more cardiovascular disease risk factors from the ACSM chart on the following page.
- ❍ You already have a known cardiovascular or pulmonary disease or a known metabolic disease, such as type 1 or type 2 diabetes; or one or more signs/symptoms that suggest any of these diseases.

ACSM Cardiovascular Disease Risk Factor Chart

❍ Family History — Myocardial infarction, coronary revascularization or sudden death before 55 years of age in father, brother, or son, or before 65 years of age in mother, sister, or daughter.

❍ Cigarette Smoking — Current smoker or quit within past 6 months

❍ High Blood Pressure — Systolic blood pressure ≥140 mm Hg or diastolic ≥90 mm Hg, confirmed by at least two separate measurements; or if you are on high blood pressure medication.

❍ High Cholesterol — Total cholesterol of >200 mg/dl or HDL of <40 mg/dl; or on lipid-lowering medication. If LDL measurement is available, use >130 mg/dl rather than total cholesterol criteria of >200 mg/dl.

❍ Impaired Fasting Glucose — Fasting blood glucose of >110 mg/dl confirmed by measurement on at least 2 separate occasions.

❍ Obesity — Body mass index of >30 or waist girth of > 88 cm for women (>102 cm for men).

❍ Sedentary Lifestyle — Not participating in a regular exercise program or meeting minimal physical activity requirements of U.S. Surgeon General's report (which is defined as accumulating 30 minutes or more of activity on most days).

(Adapted with permission from American College of Sports Medicine (2006). *ACSM's Guidelines for Exercise Testing and Prescription* (7th Ed.) Philadelphia: Lippincott Williams & Wilkins.)

Even given the above, in most cases, your doctor is still going to be in favor of you beginning an exercise program. He or she may, however, have specific recommendations for you and/or may want to supervise your efforts more closely. Please don't let this be a deterrent to getting started. Your body needs to exercise! You'll be glad you followed up.

A Few Extra Tips

- ✔ Get good shoes. You need adequate arch support, cushioning, and stability in your athletic shoes. When you are serious about fitness, treat your feet right to avoid injuries.

- ✔ Get proper instruction. This book contains detailed recommendations for many exercise options, however, if you have any questions about what is right and appropriate for you, please consult with a fitness trainer. He or she can make sure that you are performing all of your exercises properly so that you don't injure yourself and are gaining the most benefits.

- ✔ Listen to your body. Exercise should not hurt. All exercises are not right for all people. If something hurts or doesn't feel comfortable, that's your cue to stop. Pushing yourself is expected, but when your body says, "Enough," you should listen.

- ✔ Have fun! Remember, as you try to decide what is going to be the right exercise plan for you, if it isn't fun, chances are you won't be able to stick with it. We're trying to build a lifestyle that includes fitness. What can you see as part of your life?

• SECTION THREE •
The Busy Mom's Exercise Levels

Chapter 10

You've Got Lots of Options

How Much of What and When

The next question becomes, "How much of what and when?" You should have a lot of ideas percolating by now. In the following chapters, I'll give you a variety of scenarios from which to choose. You may end up concocting your own program after checking out the options in this book. I'd take that as the ultimate compliment! Remember, the name of the game is finding *your solution* – the framework that's going to get you active over the long term. Every busy mom can find some form and amount of exercise that will fit her busy schedule. It doesn't have to be a full-fledged routine, but it does have to be consistent. Slow and steady wins the race. Let's take a look at some of your options.

If placing a framework around your efforts is the path to consistency, let's divide your options into the following levels, starting with a minimalist approach all the way up to the most comprehensive plan. We'll devote an entire chapter to each level. By the end, you should see yourself fitting into one of them as your *base style*. This is the Busy Mom's Exercise Level that you think best fits your schedule, frame of mind, and goals right now.

Busy Mom's Exercise Levels:

- **The Busy Mom's "I'm Not Going To Change Into Exercise Clothes" Plan**
- **The Busy Mom's Beginner Exercise Plan**
- **The Busy Mom's Intermediate Exercise Plan**
- **The Busy Mom's Advanced Exercise Plan**

The Busy Mom's Exercise Levels are Fluid

One of the most important concepts of the Busy Mom's Exercise Levels is that they are fluid. They are not meant to put you in a box and keep you there. In fact, I had a difficult time deciding what to name the different levels because I wanted to minimize the possibility of pre-conceived judgments being attached to what level you think you "should" be at. I settled on the tried-and-true terms of beginner, intermediate, and advanced in order to clearly illustrate the progressive nature of the content. And, I felt it was completely necessary to add a level at the beginning for the busy mom who is not going to change into exercise clothes. You know who you are and you are not off the hook! I would still like you to commit to the terms outlined in that section. At any rate, the different categories are meant to represent varying levels of commitment, time, and interest, with *no judgment attached.* Choosing the Busy Mom's Beginner Exercise Plan, for instance, simply means that an honest assessment of your time, commitment, and interest matches this plan. You don't necessarily ever have to graduate to the next level if you don't want to. You will probably find that you'll slide back and forth through the different options as your time, fitness level and enthusiasm rises . . . and falls. You may slide back and forth due to travel, the seasons, or family commitments. This shift back and forth may be over a period of weeks or months, or all in the same week. There is no rule that says you can't have one workout each week that comes from each of the categories. I'm sure you haven't forgotten our ultimate goal: *consistency*. In allowing yourself the permission to slide back and forth through these levels, you will eliminate stopping altogether as an option, and the guilt that comes with it! Take a look at the four levels illustrated as position on the dial below. Also notice that the shades of gray blend seamlessly one into the next, illustrating your opportunity to choose something *in between* the levels if you wish. Only you can decide when or if it's time for you to "turn up the dial"!

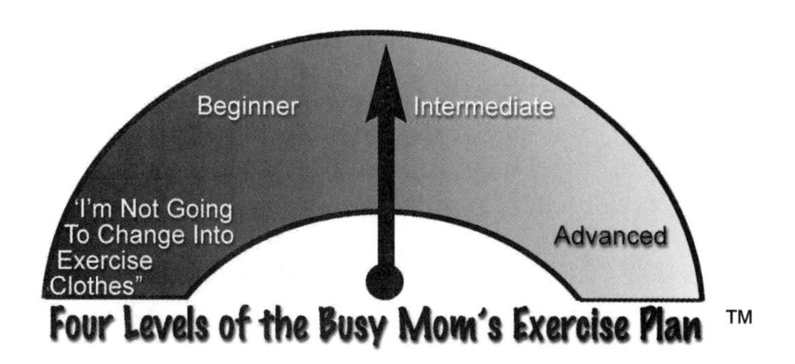

Four Levels of the Busy Mom's Exercise Plan ™

Tips for Choosing the Busy Mom's Exercise Level that is Right for You:

- ❍ Build a strong base with daily movement.
- ❍ Each level on the dial represents a progressively more comprehensive approach.
- ❍ You choose your level based on your time constraints, commitment level, and interest.
- ❍ The levels are flexible and fluid. Feel free to take it up or down a notch on the dial based on changes in your schedule and interest.
- ❍ More is better than less, but some is better than none.
- ❍ You be the judge on what level best fits you.
- ❍ Choosing none is not an option!

An Overview of the Levels

The Busy Mom's "I'm Not Going To Change Into Exercise Clothes" Plan

Accumulate 30 minutes or more of extra activity on most days.

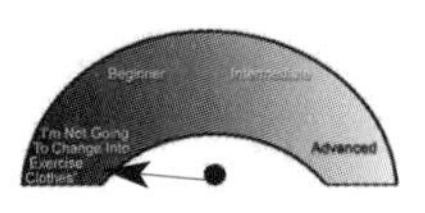

- Build it into your day, but do it consciously. Commit to several specific movement opportunities that tie into your existing lifestyle. Consider wearing a pedometer and shooting for 10,000 steps per day.

In Between?

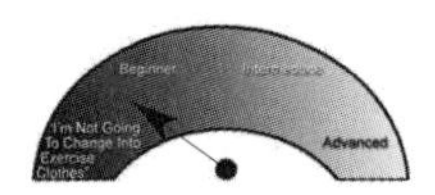

Why not take a deliberate walk for 10–15 minutes or try just the crunches or just the lower back stretch?

The Busy Mom's Beginner Exercise Plan

20 minutes of intentional exercise, 3 times per week

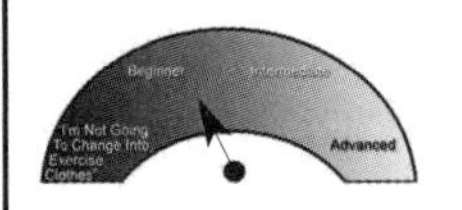

- 15 minutes of walking (you can start and end right at your own front door)
- Crunches (abdominal strengthening exercise)
- Lower back stretch

In Between?

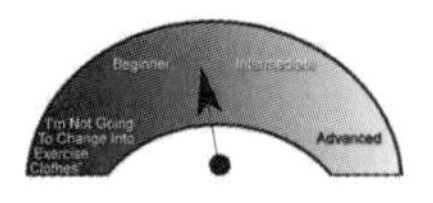

The Beginner Plan includes strengthening for only one muscle group — the abdominal muscles. The Intermediate Plan includes strengthening for all muscle groups. How about taking a look at the Intermediate Plan and adding one additional muscle group to each workout on a rotational basis?

The Busy Mom's Intermediate Exercise Plan

40 minutes of intentional exercise, 3–4 times per week

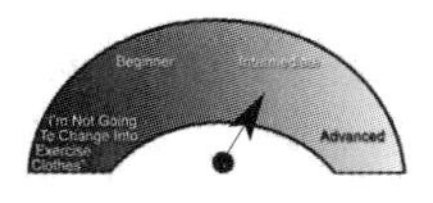

- 20 minutes of varied aerobic exercise, 3–4 times per week (walking, jogging, step aerobics, elliptical machine, stationary bicycle, etc.)
- A short (<20 minute) weight-training routine, 3 times per week (one set of one exercise per muscle group)
- Four stretching exercises for key muscle groups

In Between?

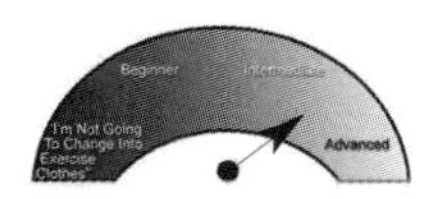

There's no reason why you can't do just one set per muscle group when you're short on time or feeling lazy and do 2–3 sets on days when you have more time or energy.

The Busy Mom's Advanced Exercise Plan

Up to 60 minutes of intentional exercise, 3–5 times per week

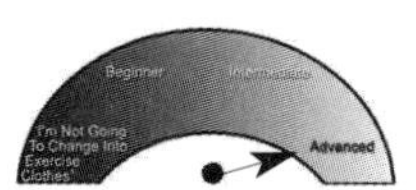

- 20–60 minutes of varied aerobic exercise, 3–5 times per week (walking, jogging, step aerobics, elliptical machine, stationary bicycle, etc.)
- A 20–40 minute weight-training routine, 3 times per week (2–3 sets per muscle group)
- Stretching exercises for each major muscle group

Where Am I Going to Do This So-Called Exercise Routine?

Little by little, we'll address exercising at home, joining a health club, as well as other creative options. Let's take it one step at a time and see what interests you and what makes sense for your lifestyle. Many successful busy mom exercisers have more than one place that they exercise and/or routines that they follow in a typical week. When they look at the big picture — it works!

What Am I Going To Use to Do This So-Called Exercise Routine?

You may also be wondering about machines vs. free weights, bands vs. balls, treadmills vs. exercise classes. We'll cover it all, one step at a time.

Where Do I Go from Here?

Remember that a fit lifestyle is progressive. By the end of this section, we'll talk about what to do when you're ready for more or ready for a change. After all, if there's no finish line, you'll need to keep your interest up and your ideas flowing.

Chapter 11

The Busy Mom's "I'm Not Going to Change into Exercise Clothes" Plan

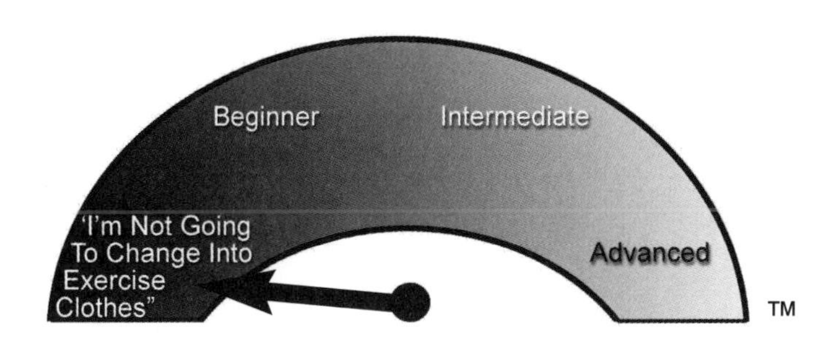

For many years, I have been using the phrase "bare minimum" to describe an exercise attitude that many people can relate to. I first started using this terminology when I was working in corporate wellness and was surrounded by very busy corporate types who wanted to gain some of the benefits of fitness . . . but didn't have a lot of time to dedicate to the proposition. They wanted to improve their health but had no grand aspirations to be the next hard-body poster child. They led busy lives and truly wanted to do the *bare minimum* necessary to gain some health benefits from physical activity. Most of them weren't quite so direct with their desire to do very little. They'd mostly hem and haw and beat around the bush until one day, someone said it flat out, "Look, I know I need to exercise. I don't have time to do much. I don't want to do much. Can you just give me the *bare minimum* I need to get by, so that I can feel good that I'm doing my duty and finally taking care of this major 'should' in my life?"

Many busy people avoid consulting with fitness professionals in the first place because they're too embarrassed to admit to someone whose life revolves around fitness that they don't really care about this stuff all *that* much. They worry that they'll end up with a time-consuming, unrealistic exercise plan that they know full well they'll never follow through with, plus a generous helping of even more guilt that they're not taking care of their bodies the way they "should." All they really wanted was a modest little program so they can check it off their list and be able to say to themselves, *"Yes, I'm addressing this area of my life."* Their goals and approach were (and are) valid, meaningful, and worthwhile. It was my job to assure these people that yes, a minimalist exercise approach is both possible and valuable . . . and then teach them how to put it into practice.

Over the next several years, the *bare minimum* became one of my most popular seminar themes and a useful approach for many of my beginner clients. And it worked. The key was *giving yourself permission* to take a modest, bare minimum approach. The collective sigh of relief was palpable.

"More may be better than less, but some is better than none."

The above phrase is the mantra of the bare minimum. Think back to the guiding theme of the first section of this book: What's going to make this time different? I'm challenging you to let go of your perfectionist, all-or-none approach, and decide that there is indeed a middle ground. You know yourself. You probably know whether you are in a place and time that'll make a comprehensive fitness program realistic or not. If not, it's time to let go of the black and white and find what will give you some of the wonderful benefits, but on your terms. Remember the sneaky observation I made previously in Section One? When you start with a minimalist program, it often grows and turns into something more substantial over time. And, all the while, you are still doing something wonderful for your health!

So, what's the Busy Mom's "I'm Not Going to Change into Exercise Clothes" Plan all about? I like to call this Busy Mom's Exercise Level, "Daily Activity Adds Up," because the goal is simply to add more activity to your existing daily life, and because it truly does add up!

You are perfect for this Busy Mom's Exercise Level if:

- You feel "allergic to exercise" — don't like it, never did, and don't see it changing anytime soon.
- You've never liked to sweat.
- You can't see where or how you'd set aside a specific recurring time to exercise.
- You don't really want to set aside a specific recurring time to exercise.
- You don't see yourself changing into exercise clothes to work out.

Does this sound like you? The Busy Mom's "I'm Not Going to Change into Exercise Clothes" Plan is for every busy mom who has never thought of herself as being into fitness, but who can no longer ignore all the benefits of exercise. Just because you're not the exercise-type doesn't mean you should let yourself off the hook altogether. So, here we have the perfect compromise! Also remember, you're looking for what describes you right now. Keep in mind that you may grow out of this stage. Whether you do or whether you don't, it's not a bad place to be, as long as you make the most of it.

Here's the goal of the Busy Mom's "I'm Not Going to Change into Exercise Clothes" Plan:

Accumulate 30 minutes of extra activity on most days.

The goal of the Busy Mom's "I'm Not Going to Change into Exercise Clothes" Plan is to accumulate 30 minutes of extra activity on most days. It doesn't have to be all at once. It can be interspersed throughout the day. That's it. Sound too simple? Sound too insignificant? Think again. Let's bring alive all the benefits of adopting this way of life and then get to the tips that will make it happen. And while you consider how *daily activity adds up,* let me add that this way of life is beneficial for all busy moms, even those who are also incorporating more rigorous exercise routines on top of increasing daily activity.

Daily Activity Adds Up

We all know that it is good to be more active rather than less active. Our bodies thrive on movement, yet many of us spend just a few too many hours in front of the TV or computer. When we do think about activity, most of us think automatically about structured exercise — the kind that is on purpose, while wearing exercise clothing . . . the kind that we don't have time for.

Think again — this time about the little things that make up an active lifestyle and *make a difference!* You know those tips such as "park farther away" or "take the stairs instead of the elevator"? If you're like most people, you may agree that it sounds good, but are secretly thinking, "That stuff can't possibly make a difference." Guess again! "That stuff" *does* make a difference. And here's why:

Our bodies are calorie-burning machines 24 hours a day. Even if you exercised one full hour per day (which is a *lot*), there are still 23 hours of metabolic activity to be accounted for. If you don't give a second thought to your activity level throughout the day, you are missing a great opportunity to have a huge impact on your health and your weight. What is *your* body doing the other twenty-three hours per day?

All in a Day's Work . . . or Lack-There-Of

You may remember from the chapter on resistance training that the average busy mom burns approximately one calorie per minute, sitting at rest. The same busy mom, while standing, will burn *1.5* calories per minute. You may be thinking "an extra half calorie . . . big deal". Now, while it may be small potatoes for one minute, or even one hour, *50% more calories to stand vs. sit* is a pretty big deal when you spend a good part of your day sitting vs. standing!

Walking at a leisurely pace burns approximately two calories per minute — *double* that of sitting! Aerobic exercise, such as brisk walking, jogging, etc. can burn up to 8–12 calories per minute. That's why aerobic exercise is a great way to burn a nice extra chunk of calories per day and can help with weight loss. But, since aerobic exercise isn't realistically going to account for a very big part of your day, it's a good idea to give some thought to the daily activities that make up the other 23 hours of the day. They truly add up!

While I was in graduate school, we had to do an experiment that highlighted how inactive many of us are without even realizing it. The task involved keeping a log of our activity level in 15-minute intervals for an entire 24-hour period. (24 hours multiplied by 4 entries per hour = 96 entries into the log!) We assigned a code to each 15-minute interval according to the following: 1 = lying down or sleeping, 2 = sitting, 3 = standing, 4 = walking, 5 = higher level of exercise. Once we had the numeric codes for each 15-minute interval, we could calculate an estimate of how many calories we burned in that day. Of course, as exercise physiology students, we were all pretty confident that we would fare well in the experiment. As it turned out, none of us were as active as we thought. It was an eye-opening (not to mention humbling) experience to see a page full of 1s and 2s! Many of us gave more thought to our daily activity after that.

And the Days Turn into Weeks

Let's take it one step further to give some thought to your metabolic activity in an entire week. There are 168 hours in a week. Using our example of a busy mom who exercises for a full hour each day, there are still another 161 hours (or 96%) of the week to consider! Can you think of any other area in your life in which you'd like to make an improvement and chose to ignore 96% of the time available to you?

Remember the section early on about "The World We Live In"? Keep in mind how our labor-and time-saving culture robs us of opportunities to use our bodies. Think drive-thru fast food, circling for the closest spot (even if it takes longer), waiting and waiting for the elevator instead of taking the stairs, ride-on lawn mowers and self-propelled vacuum cleaners, and emailing someone sitting in the cube down the hall. Physical labor used to be part of the average American's day, but it is no more. You can turn that around! Choose the more active option rather than the less active option. Seek out ways to use your body rather than ways to save energy.

But I Never Sit Down!

Most of the busy moms I know are already moving a lot throughout the day, but there are exceptions. You may be a busy working mom — lots on your mental to-do list, and lots of activity after work and on the weekends, but a whole lot of sitting between the hours of nine to five. Or maybe you're a stay-at-home or work-from-home busy mom who is sitting a little more often than she realizes.

Taking Action

Armed with the reasons why, let's take another look at the tried-and-true suggestions below. I like to think of these techniques as "sneaking exercise" into your day. They are all little things that separately seem insignificant, but together, can make a big difference.

- Stand rather than sit when you can.
- Take the stairs instead of the elevator.
- Park at the far end of the parking lot.
- Get off the metro one stop early and walk the rest of the distance.

- ❖ Stand up while talking on the phone.
- ❖ Walk down the hall at the office to deliver a message in person.
- ❖ When straightening up the house, go up and down the stairs as you go rather than making a big pile at the bottom of the stairs to bring up in one trip later.
- ❖ Get down on the floor and play with your children.
- ❖ If you have older children, take a bike ride or go for a walk.

Make It Real; Make It a Conscious Decision

So, even if you are already moving around a good bit during the day, it might not be real or quantifiable or on-purpose enough for your health. Why not try to take it to that next level? Here are some ideas for holding yourself accountable for your goal of accumulating thirty minutes or more of activity on most days. It will seem more concrete if you make specific decisions and try to reset your patterns. Vague rarely works. Get specific and you'll see things happen. Which of the following thought patterns do you think will most likely lead to success?

"I'm going to try to take the stairs more often instead of the elevator."

"I will take the stairs Monday through Friday when I go to the cafeteria at lunchtime."

How about these two choices?

"I'm going to try to walk more often throughout the day."

"Every time I go shopping, I'll park at the far end of the lot to make for a longer walk to the front door."

Make a Plan

Break up the 30 minutes into three 10-minute exercise bites throughout the day. Find some small way to increase the movement involved in something that's already part of your morning, afternoon, and/or evening routine. Maybe you'll take a quick trip around the block after you wave goodbye to the school bus in the morning if you're a stay-at-home mom. Maybe you'll go for another mini-walk after dinner every evening. Nothing hard core, but intentional. That's the difference.

Use a Pedometer

Pedometers are awesome! You can see that specific goals make this technique come to life. Here's another great way to get you more conscious of how much you move throughout the day. A pedometer is a simple little device, that when clipped to the waistband of your clothing, counts how many steps you take. The fancier pedometers also track total distance covered in miles or kilometers, total calories burned and lots of other interesting facts. You can find pedometers at any sporting goods store or order one from www.busymomsolutions.com.

The Surgeon General's "Shape Up America" Program (www.shapeup.org) recommends the goal of taking 10,000 steps per day.

Ten thousand steps, you say?! That does sound like an awful lot. The first step is to get your pedometer. Next, you will just wear it for a few days to a week without changing your habits at all. This will give you a good idea of how many steps you take when you're not even trying to be more active. Let's say that you find that you are averaging approximately 3,000 steps a day. Does 10,000 steps seem pretty far off? Maybe so — at first. The key will be to gradually build it up. Week by week, you can set a goal of averaging 500 steps a day more than the week before. Remember, we're trying to set some long-term habits. There's no need to rush into anything. You will find over time that you'll need to do some conscious activity to get up to 10,000 steps a day. But my promise to you was that you don't necessarily need to change into exercise clothes to do it. Go for a walk? Yes. Change into exercise clothes for a "power walk"? No. Build some new small habits into your day — take a quick walk with the stroller or ban yourself from the elevator at work and see what happens to the numbers. There may be other activities that you enjoy that get you moving. Get creative and keep wearing the pedometer for a while. Raising your consciousness is what's going to make the difference. Once you get into the habit, there may come a time when you find you don't need to wear it to approximate your activity anymore. Success!

The Benefits

So what are the benefits of trying to accumulate 30 minutes of activity or 10,000 steps a day?

There are *phenomenal long-term health benefits* in your future if you adopt this lifestyle, including:

- Improved general health.
- Increased energy.
- Reduced risk of a host of chronic diseases — heart disease, diabetes, and some cancers.
- Increased calorie burning from more activity.
- A positive experience of not biting off more than you can chew and getting burned out.
- Consistency with an intentional effort toward fitness.
- A fitness-conscious mindset that may lead to a lifetime of exercise!

As wonderful as these benefits are, this level of exercise will not translate into large gains in traditional fitness benefits, such as aerobic capacity and muscular strength. Those benefits increase substantially with the next level. Who knows? You may be there soon!

Tips on Using a Pedometer

- ▲ Use the number of steps recorded only as a gauge of your overall activity level and to compare one day to the next. Your pedometer may not be extremely accurate in capturing exactly how many steps you take. (For instance, if you walk 10 paces, your pedometer may register 8–14 steps.) You will still be able to tell if your activity level increases or decreases from day to day.
- ▲ Find a pedometer that has a comfortable, yet secure way to attach to your clothing. Some even come with a short tether to keep them secure.
- ▲ Even if you never get near 10,000 steps per day, a pedometer can still be useful. There is much to be gained from increasing your day-to-day movement even just a little. Another non-profit organization, America On the Move™, (www.americaonthemove.org) recommends you use a pedometer to see how many steps you average each day and set a goal of increasing it by 2,000 steps per day. You may find this goal to be more realistic for you than 10,000 steps per day. *Good luck and have fun with it!*

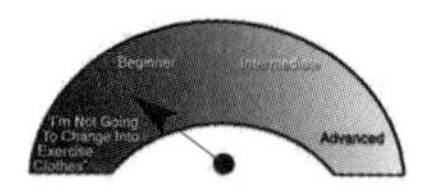

Ready for a Little More?

Why not take a deliberate walk for 10 or 15 minutes? You could also take a look at the crunches and lower back stretch in the Busy Mom's Beginner Exercise Plan. You might want to try one or both of them, even if it's not on a consistent basis.

Increased Daily Activity Is Great For Every Busy Mom

Increased daily movement or 10,000 steps a day is great for every busy mom, not just the "I'm Not Going to Change into Exercise Clothes" set. Are you a busy mom who is also planning on doing some exercise on purpose, in exercise clothing? You, too, can benefit from increasing your activity throughout the day. It's not an either-or proposition. Please join us!

Chapter 12

The Busy Mom's Beginner Exercise Plan

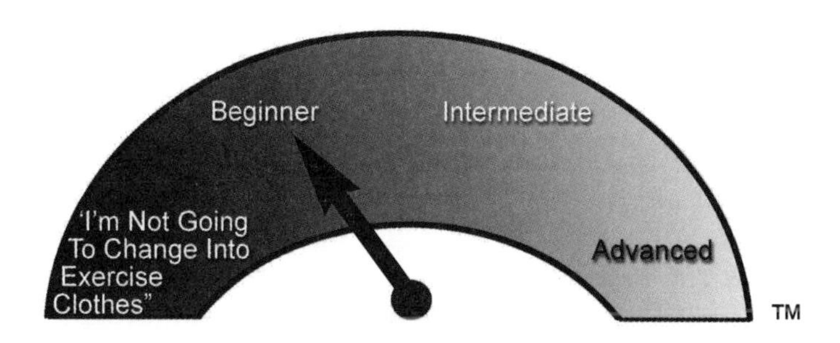

Okay, you've decided that you'd like to commit to exercising on purpose several times per week, but still think a minimalist approach is the way to go, at least for now. Bravo! You'll need to commit to the following schedule:

20 minutes of intentional exercise all at once, 3 times per week

- 15 minutes of walking
- Crunches (abdominal strengthening exercise)
- Lower back stretch

Why did I select these particular exercises? In just 20 minutes of intentional exercise, these particular exercises will allow you to do something that addresses each of the three categories of exercise: aerobic exercise, resistance training, and stretching. Is it the "be-all, end-all" for each category? Of course not. We are talking about the bare minimum for an intentional exercise session. A mini-aerobic workout and hitting one or two muscle groups is better than nothing and has much to offer. If you only have time to strengthen one muscle group, the abdominal muscles get my vote. Strengthening your abdominal muscles and stretching your lower back muscles go together like peanut butter and jelly. Popular fitness lingo these days refers to these muscle groups as part of your "core," meaning that their conditioning impacts your body's overall stability and ability to comfortably do lots of other things. Strong abdominal muscles help with posture, prevent lower back pain, and can improve your appearance. (Taut abdominal muscles hold all your internal organs in nice and tight, giving you a more slender appearance from the side view.) Lower back muscle stretching is one of the simplest stretching exercises to perform correctly without much instruction. It has wonderful benefits for alleviating or preventing lower back pain, especially when combined with crunches. Walking is the simplest form of aerobic exercise. Sure, you can do it at a health club or on a treadmill at home if you choose, but more importantly, it can start and end at your own front door. No financial investment necessary, no special equipment necessary. (You should however, invest in a good pair of walking shoes at some point, if you're serious.) The walking will build a base of aerobic exercise that you can build on if you choose. After all, once you start walking, you may decide to go longer than 15 minutes. But, you tell yourself that you only need to go for 15 minutes and consider your goal accomplished if you complete it. Your crunches and lower back stretch should take an additional 5 minutes. This is a perfectly respectable exercise program. Don't forget to congratulate yourself!

The Benefits

Look at all you will be doing for yourself by adopting this level of exercise:

- ✔ All of the benefits listed in the Busy Mom's "I'm Not Going to Change into Exercise Clothes" Plan
  - ❖ Improved general health.
  - ❖ Increased energy.
  - ❖ Reduced risk of a host of chronic diseases — heart disease, diabetes, and some cancers.
  - ❖ Increased calorie burning from more activity.
  - ❖ A positive experience of not biting off more than you can chew and getting burned out.
  - ❖ Consistency with an intentional effort toward fitness.
  - ❖ A fitness-conscious mindset that may lead to a lifetime of exercise!

Plus:

- ✔ Improved strength and capacity of your heart and lungs.
- ✔ Improved blood pressure.
- ✔ Increased muscular endurance and tone in your legs.
- ✔ An outlet for stress.
- ✔ Improved sleep patterns.
- ✔ Stronger and more taut abdominal muscles leading to improved appearance.
- ✔ Alleviation or prevention of lower back pain.
- ✔ A sense of accomplishment and possibly a hankering for more exercise down the road?

Getting Started Tips

Before you begin, it's a great idea to decide the usual days and times that you are going to do your new exercise routine. If you leave it vague as to which days of the week you'll exercise, it often doesn't happen. If you say to yourself, "I'll do my routine every Monday, Wednesday, and Saturday morning," you'll stand a better chance of doing it consistently. Actually write it into your schedule? Even better. Sure, you'll switch days or times on occasion, but that'll be the exception, rather than the norm.

Fitness Walking Tips

Start and End at a Comfortable Pace

Be sure to warm-up and cool-down by simply walking at a slower pace during the first and last few minutes of your walk. The warm-up gradually prepares your body for exercise and the cool-down gradually brings your heart rate back to normal.

Watch Your Intensity

The goal in exercise walking is "brisk." It shouldn't feel like a stroll, but it also shouldn't feel "really hard" either. A moderate, "somewhat hard" pace is the goal – one you can maintain for at least 15 minutes. The "Talk Test" is a good measure of intensity if you don't want to bother with the other methods outlined in Chapter Six. If you can't talk while walking, you're working too hard. If you could gab continuously, however, you're probably not working hard enough!

Measure a Course . . . Or Not

Some people prefer to walk at a nearby track or on a measured route in order to determine how far they walk. Others prefer the simplicity of just starting and ending at their own front door. The choice is yours!

Keep It Up

Make walking a part of your daily activities. Put it into your schedule. Pick a time that is best for you. Enlist a friend to be a walking partner. Go to the mall on bad weather days. Vary the course to make it interesting. Consistency is always the goal!

When You're Ready to Up the Ante

If you've been at it for a while and would like to step things up a notch, try adding some hills into your course or try "interval walking." With intervals, you sprinkle short bursts of a faster pace into your regular walk. These bursts can be a minute long or even less. They don't have to be structured, either. You may want to challenge yourself to "walk as fast as you can" to the next tree or telephone pole, perhaps, and then bring it back to your normal pace. A few minutes later, you may repeat the challenge.

How to Walk

It may sound odd to need instruction on "how" to walk. But when you're walking for exercise, it's important to know about correct posture, arm swing, and stride length.

Posture

Your whole body should lean slightly forward from the ankles. (Don't lean from the waist. This will make your back tired and breathing more difficult.) Keep your head and chin up, shoulders relaxed and pulled back, and your abdominal muscles tightened for good back support. (Sounds like a lot to think about? Try thinking about one or two tips at a time.)

Arm Swing

Try to keep your elbows bent at about a 90-degree angle or whatever is most comfortable for you. Swing from the shoulder, not the elbow. Your hands should not swing higher than chest level during the forward swing. Keep your arms close to your body and parallel to your body. If you use the 90-degree arm swing, you will burn 5–10% more calories than just allowing your arms to swing naturally without thinking about it. However, it's not for everyone. You may feel awkward doing so, or just prefer not to. That's fine!

Stride

Avoid the tendency to take longer strides to go faster. Unlike runners, walkers need to move their feet faster by taking more steps per minute while maintaining their natural stride. With each step, your heel should strike the ground first, then roll through the ball of your foot and push off from the toe.

A Quick Stretch at the End

A quick calf stretch at the end of your walk is a good idea, especially if your pace is brisk. It's not the end of the world if you skip it, but read the following so at least you'll know what it is, should you choose to add it in:

Standing Calf Stretch

Stand with your feet together and simply take a big step backward with one foot. Next, shift your weight forward so that your front knee is bent, but the knee is not jutting out past your toes. Be sure to keep the heel of your back foot on the floor. If you don't feel a stretch in your calf (of the back leg), you'll need to take a bigger step backwards with the back leg. Simply hold this position for about 15 seconds and then switch.

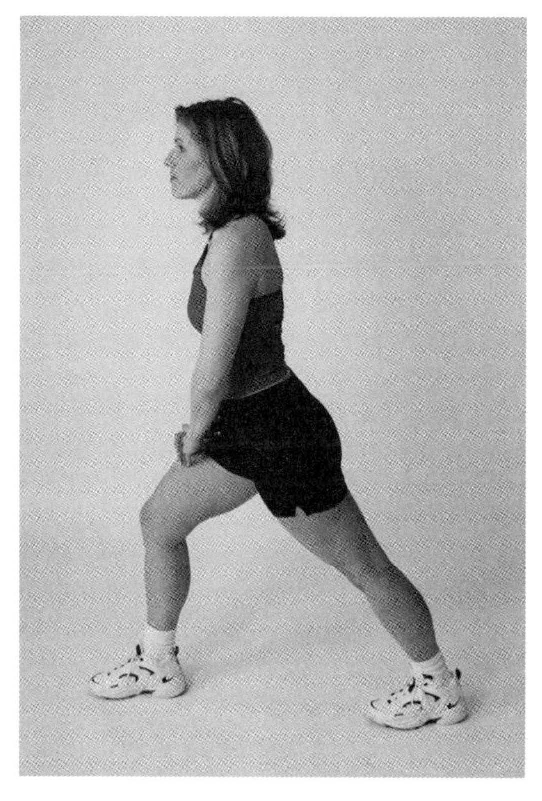

Standing Calf Stretch

Goodbye Back Pain and Hello Strong, Taut Mid-Section

Do you suffer from occasional lower back pain? Did you know that many cases of lower back pain are actually caused by weak *abdominal muscles?* That's right – weak, sagging abdominal muscles can tug the pelvis forward and down, tilting it. This forward pelvic tilt can make the lower back muscles tighten, when what you want is for them to be stretched and relaxed.

How to reverse it? That's simple! To tilt the pelvis *back* into alignment, you need to follow a two-part formula:

1) Strengthen the abdominal muscles
2) Stretch the lower back muscles

To strengthen the abdominal muscles, start with basic crunches:

The Crunch

Lie on the floor on your back, with your knees bent and your feet flat on the floor. Your hands can be either crossed over your chest or placed lightly behind your head (not behind your neck). Slowly lift your head and shoulders off the floor until you feel your shoulder blades come off the floor, and then slowly return to the starting position. Be sure to keep your head and neck relaxed during the movement – don't jut your chin up toward the ceiling OR tuck your chin to your chest. Just allow it to remain neutral and natural as you curl up and down. How many crunches should you do? That will depend directly on how strong your abdominal muscles are! You may start with 5, 10, 20 or even 50 crunches! See how you feel and stop when your stomach muscles feel fatigued. Over a period of time, you will be able to do more and more crunches. That will also tell you that you may be ready for more advanced abdominal strengthening exercises!

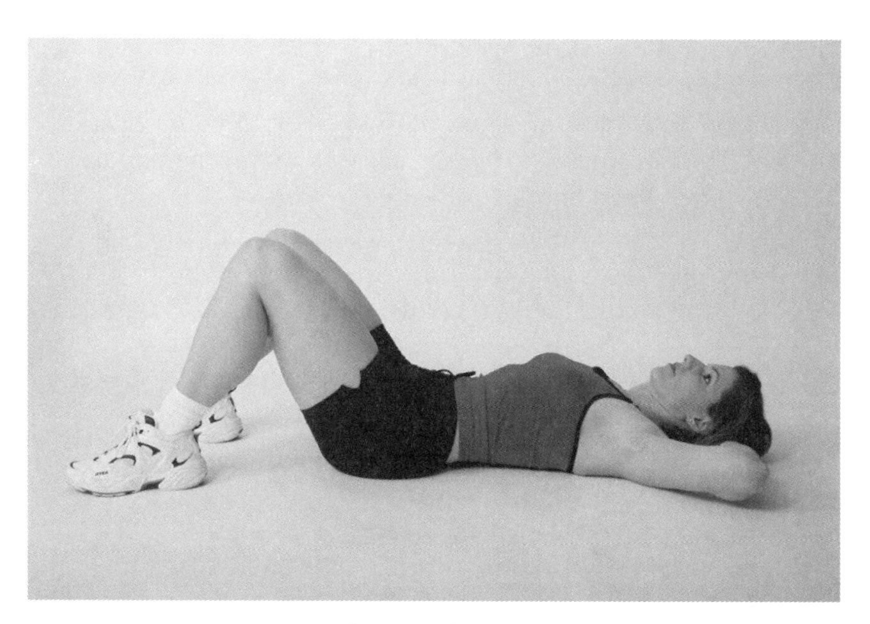

The Crunch (start)

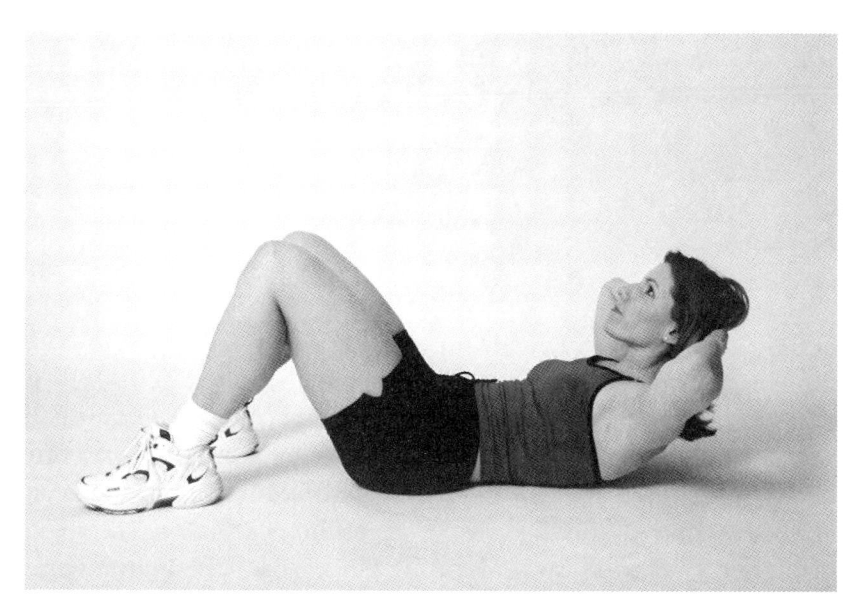

The Crunch (finish)

Lower Back Stretch

Lie on your back and pull both knees into your chest. Hold both knees to your chest with your hands, clasping your hands under your knees if possible. Hold this position for at least 30 seconds, or as long as 3 minutes if you have chronic lower back pain. If you can only hold it for 30 seconds, repeat it several times.

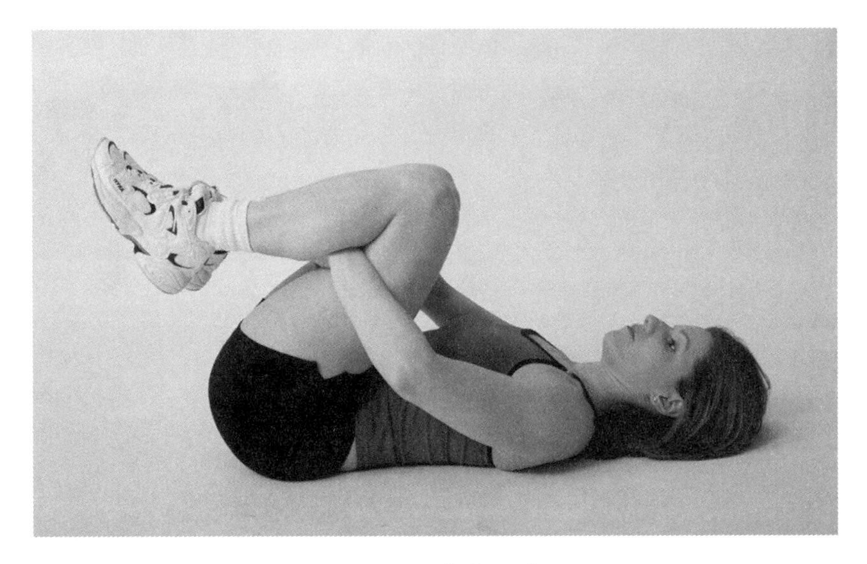

Lower Back Stretch

Putting It Together

Do these two exercises together, which makes sense since the starting position is the same (lying on the floor on your back). You can either do the crunches first and the lower back stretch second OR do the lower back stretch before *and* after the crunches. While the Busy Mom's Beginner Exercise Plan recommends that you do this routine 3 times per week, crunches and the lower back stretch are mild enough that you can do them more frequently, even every day, if you'd like.

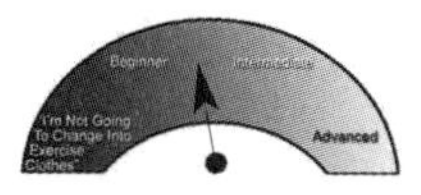

Looking for a Little More?

Remember, the Busy Mom's Exercise Levels blend seamlessly together on a progressive path. Would you like to try out some of the other muscle strengthening exercises in addition to the crunches, but don't want to commit to doing all of them every time you workout?

There is a great middle ground that will give you a taste of a slightly more comprehensive approach to resistance training without adding much time to your regular workout. Here's how it works. For each workout, simply complete your 15 minutes of walking, plus your crunches and the lower back stretch. Then, add one additional resistance training exercise – picking a different muscle group each time.

Simply refer to Appendix 2 for the listing of additional resistance training exercises for you to choose from. In the intermediate plan, you go through all the major muscle groups each time you workout. (You'll recall that hitting each muscle group three times per week is the *best* way to get a muscle stronger and firmer.) But if you are interested in picking a different muscle group to hit with every workout, in addition to your abdominal muscles, each major muscle group will have some stimulus every now and then. It's a great bridge between the beginner and intermediate levels. You'll gain knowledge and experience with what exercises work each muscle group, making for an easy transition to the Busy Mom's Intermediate Exercise Plan, should you decide to do that at some point.

Remember, the benefits aren't always just physiological, and you are on a lifetime journey. Don't be too quick to discount working each muscle group only occasionally just because the official guidelines are to do resistance training for each muscle group three times each week. If you're a busy mom who doesn't see that happening anytime soon, you can still do a little and benefit from it. Congratulations!

Chapter 13

The Busy Mom's Intermediate Exercise Plan

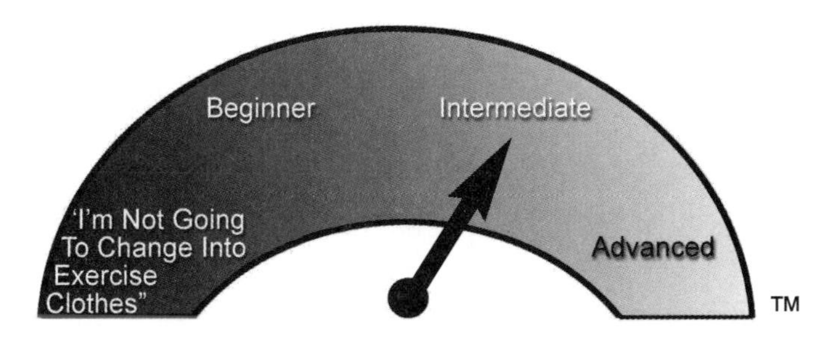

We are getting into the meat and potatoes now! The Busy Mom's Intermediate Exercise Plan is my favorite busy mom's exercise level! It delivers great benefits, but is still realistic for your busy schedule. Here's how it works:

40 minutes of intentional exercise, 3–4 times per week

- 20 minutes of varied aerobic exercise, 3–4 times per week (walking, jogging, step aerobics, elliptical machine, stationary bicycle, etc.)
- A short (<20 minute) weight-training routine, 3 times per week (one set of one exercise per muscle group)
- Four stretching exercises for key muscle groups

Did you notice that the Busy Mom's Intermediate Exercise Plan lists aerobic activity 3-4 times per week and weight training only 3 times per week? The fourth aerobic session is a "bonus" — if you can do it, great and you'll reap even more benefits. But if not, that's fine, too! Many busy moms will prefer to schedule themselves three 40-minute timeslots per week to do both their aerobic activity and their weight training one after the other. If it's easier on your schedule to break them up, that's fine, too.

Let's look at the specifics for each of these components.

20 Minutes of Aerobic Activity

The Busy Mom's Beginner Exercise Plan recommends walking as the form of aerobic activity because it is simple and easily accessible for almost all busy moms. When you are ready to step things up to the Busy Mom's Intermediate Exercise Plan, you might want to mix up the walking with other modes of aerobic activity, although you can certainly keep it to just walking if that's what's best for you. In addition, going from 15 to 20 minutes for your aerobic workout gets you into the gold standard "20 minutes or more" recommendations by ACSM for cardiovascular exercise.

What are the choices for aerobic activity?

★ Walking (on a treadmill or outside)

★ Jogging (on a treadmill or outside)

  Jogging may very well be too intense for you. If it interests you, start with sprinkling little spurts of a slow jog into your walking. You might start with 4 or 5 minutes of walking for each 1 minute of jogging. Little by little, increase the amount of time you spend jogging and decrease the amount of time you spend walking. Make sure it's gradual and fun, if you choose to do so.

- ★ Any aerobic exercise equipment that you find at a health club or that you can buy for home use:
  - Stair climber machine
  - Elliptical trainer machine
  - Stationary bicycle
  - Cross country ski machine
  - A mini-trampoline
- ★ Swimming
- ★ A step aerobics class or any other class listed as "cardio"
- ★ Any exercise videotape that lists "aerobic workout" or "cardiovascular workout" as the type

A Short Weight-training Routine

As a starting point, this routine is designed as something that you can do at home. If you end up joining a club of some kind, your options for how to work each muscle group increase. At that point, you'll begin thinking in terms of hitting each muscle group, rather than following a set list of exercises. You'll slowly learn several exercises for each muscle group, and can begin to vary which exercise you do for each muscle group. We'll cover those types of options in the Busy Mom's Advanced Exercise Plan, although you may very well begin to vary your exercises while still doing an intermediate level exercise routine.

If you've made the mental leap to the Busy Mom's Intermediate Exercise Plan, you won't mind me saying that it's time to invest in a few pieces of inexpensive exercise equipment in order to work each muscle group more effectively. You can find everything in the fitness section of many large retail stores, in addition to any sports store, online fitness outlets, and at my site, www.busymomsolutions.com.

Here's your shopping list:

- ❍ **Two or Three Pairs of Dumbbells**

  You'll need two or three pairs of dumbbells because you'll be able to handle more weight for exercises that target larger muscle groups, while needing smaller weights for exercises that target smaller muscle groups or are otherwise harder for you. Remember from the chapter on resistance training that for each exercise *you're looking for a weight that causes you to reach fatigue by 8–15 repetitions at the most.* That means that you can't keep going. Many women make the mistake of using dumbbells that are entirely too light. One and 2-pound dumbbells are generally only appropriate in rehabilitation or geriatric settings. I'm pretty sure most busy moms can handle at least 3-pound dumbbells! For many, even 3-pounders will be too light. Many busy moms will need 5-, 8-, and 10-pound dumbbells, while others may not need 5 pounders at all, and may need 8-, 10-, and 12- or even 15- or 20-pound dumbbells. (Yes, I did say 15- and 20-pound dumbbells!) You'll be surprised what you'll be able to do before long. Keep in mind that as your strength increases, you'll graduate to larger dumbbells over time. An ideal situation would be one in which you could try out each exercise with different size dumbbells before you buy them so that you know what sizes you'll need.

- ❍ **Exercise Tubing with Handles**

  Dumbbells are great for many exercises, but not all, and here's why. Dumbbells give you resistance against gravity, right? (They weigh down as you try to lift them up.) If you hold them up and then try to do a horizontal movement, the muscles getting most of the work are the ones holding the dumbbells up, not the muscles struggling to do a horizontal movement while in that position. Make sense? There are also muscles that are best worked doing a motion in which you pull *down*. Holding dumbbells over your head and pulling them down is *not* the right idea. What's really causing the dumbbells to come down in this scenario? Yes; gravity again. You might've hurried it up by pulling the dumbbells down, but you are not getting any muscular work by doing so. Exercise tubing is ideal for creating resistance in a horizontal plane or overhead. It's also inexpensive, versatile, and perfect for travel. (Dumbbells are never a great addition to your suitcase!) Exercise tubing comes in a variety of diameters that are usually color-coded — the thicker the tubing, the harder the resistance.

❍ **A large, lightweight, inflated exercise ball**

You've probably seen these balls, often called "stability balls." They are now so popular that you don't need to go to a sporting goods store to buy these either. There are several sizes available that correspond to your height. The most common size ball is "55 cm." As a general guideline, women on the shorter side (under 5'1") may prefer a 45 cm ball, and women over 5'9" may prefer a 65 cm ball. They are wonderfully versatile, inexpensive, and fun to use!

Where to Purchase Your Dumbbells, Exercise Tubing, and Exercise Ball

Online

For your convenience, I've set up www.busymomsolutions.com with the exact equipment that I recommend for the exercise routines found in this book. You'll be able to order exercise balls, tubing, pedometers, and more. No searching or wondering if you found the right products, and no extra errands to run. Visit me there to order your supplies and they'll be delivered right to your doorstep.

There are also many other fitness equipment websites that sell exercise balls and tubing. I would not recommend purchasing dumbbells online, however, as shipping costs are based on weight and will be quite expensive. You're better off visiting a retail location near you to purchase dumbbells.

Retail Stores

You can find dumbbells, exercise tubing, and exercise balls at your local sporting goods specialty store, as well as in the sporting goods department of many large, general retailers.

The Benefits

Onward and upward with the cumulative benefits as you work through the levels! The benefits of the Busy Mom's Intermediate Exercise Plan are truly wonderful! Take a look:

✔ All of the benefits listed in the Busy Mom's "I'm Not Going to Change into Exercise Clothes" Plan, and the Busy Mom's Beginner Exercise Plan, **but to a larger degree!** More exercise, and increased rigor of the routine will increase the level of benefit you receive from each of the following points listed. Good for you!

- ❖ Improved general health.
- ❖ Increased energy.
- ❖ Reduced risk of a host of chronic diseases — heart disease, diabetes, and some cancers.
- ❖ Increased calorie burning from more activity.
- ❖ A positive experience of not biting off more than you can chew and getting burned out.
- ❖ Consistency with an intentional effort toward fitness.
- ❖ A fitness-conscious mindset that may lead to a lifetime of exercise!
- ❖ Improved strength and capacity of your heart and lungs.
- ❖ Improved blood pressure.
- ❖ Increased muscular endurance and tone in many muscle groups from the aerobic activity.
- ❖ An outlet for stress.
- ❖ Improved sleep patterns.
- ❖ Stronger and more taut abdominal muscles leading to improved appearance.

- ❖ Alleviation or prevention of lower back pain.
- ❖ A sense of accomplishment and possibly a hankering for more exercise down the road.

Plus:

- ✔ Noticeable increased muscular strength and endurance for all of your major muscles groups!
- ✔ An even greater increase in metabolic rate!
- ✔ Even greater improvement in aerobic capacity/cardiovascular endurance!
- ✔ Help with weight loss due to more substantial increases in metabolism and calorie burning!
- ✔ Knowledge and practice in knowing what makes up a comprehensive resistance training routine, making for an easy transition to the Busy Mom's Advanced Exercise Plan, should you decide to do that at some point.

The Busy Mom's Intermediate Weight Training Routine

You'll perform one set of each of the following ten exercises. (Refer to Appendix 2 for photos and descriptions of each exercise.)

1. Dumbbell Chest Press or Pushups (chest)
2. Seated Tubing Row (back)
3. Dumbbell Side Raise (shoulders)
4. Dumbbell Bicep Curl (biceps/front of arm)
5. Overhead Tricep Extension with a Dumbbell (triceps/back of arm)
6. Ball Squat or Dumbbell Squat (quadriceps/front of thigh and gluteus maximus/rear end)
7. Ball Hamstring Curl (hamstrings/back of thigh)
8. Inner Thigh Ball Squeeze (inner thigh)
9. Hip Abduction with Tubing (hips)
10. Crunches (abdominal muscles)

This top-ten list allows you to hit every major muscle group in 20 minutes or less. Can you start with just a few and build up to all ten later? Absolutely! Can you skip a muscle group or two when you are short on time? Absolutely again! Remember, *more may be better than less, but some is better than none!*

Balance, proper form, and posture are important in doing each exercise correctly — both for maximum benefit and also for injury prevention. You'll be performing one set of 8–15 repetitions for all of the dumbbell exercises. With ball or tubing exercises, there is no way to increase the resistance, therefore, depending on your strength, you'll just do more repetitions until you reach fatigue — it could be as many as 30–50 repetitions. You probably remember from our chapter on resistance training that performing such high reps with a limited resistance isn't ideal for strength gains, but it's the best we have available for this level of commitment and in this setting. You'll still get plenty of good results as long as you continue *until your muscles feel fatigued.* Don't stop the first minute it starts to feel difficult!

The Busy Mom's Intermediate Exercise Plan Four Key Stretches

A great way to finish off your intermediate level exercise routine is with a few stretches for those major muscle groups most in need of some TLC after a workout. There are four stretches in the Busy Mom's Intermediate Exercise Plan. Each stretch is pictured and described in detail in Appendix 2. You can hold each stretch for as little as 10–15 seconds for a quick stretch, up to 30 seconds when you're relaxing a little more into the stretch, or as long as a minute or two when you are nursing a problem in that area. *Remember not to bounce.* The four stretches are:

1. Quadriceps Stretch
2. Calf Stretch
3. Lower Back Stretch
4. Hamstring Stretch

So that's the Busy Mom's Intermediate Exercise Plan. What do you think? Is it realistic for you? Yes or no, it's always here. Maybe you're beyond it and may decide to use it during a busy week when you need to scale back your normal routine, or maybe you're not up to it yet, but it's your goal for six months from now. You're not competing with anyone else and it's all good!

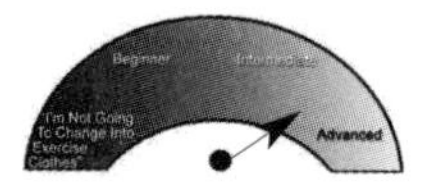

Ready for a Little More?

Why not add an extra 5–10 minutes to your cardio workout, try a second set of weights every now and then, or add a few new stretches to your routine?

Chapter 14

The Busy Mom's Advanced Exercise Plan

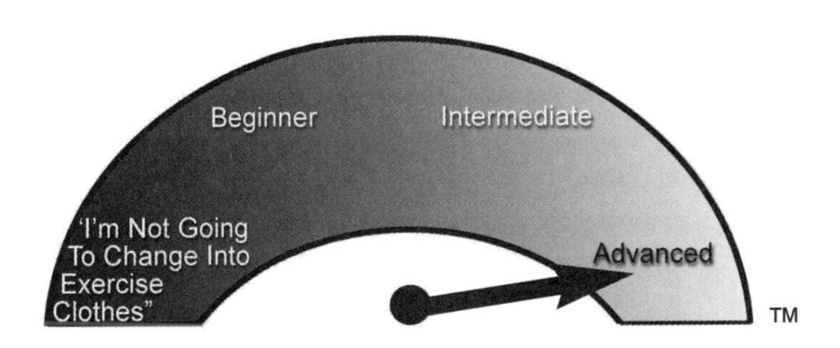

It's time to consider the Busy Mom's Advanced Exercise Plan if you're a busy mom on a roll! If this doesn't sound like where you are now, who knows, you may be re-reading this section next year and finding it fits you perfectly. The particulars of the advanced level are a great basis for comparison to the other options available. If you're an advanced gal, you may not need much guidance or motivation. Then again, there are degrees within this program, too. I know more than a few "super moms" who could benefit from new ideas about how to scale back when their normal full-fledged routine is just too much, as well as permission to do so. Once you've arrived at this level, it's time to look at all the options within it. What makes up the Busy Mom's Advanced Exercise Plan?

Up to 60 minutes of intentional exercise, 3–5 times per week

- 20–60 minutes of varied aerobic exercise, 3–5 times per week (walking, jogging, step aerobics, elliptical machine, stationary bicycle, etc.)
- A 20–40 minute weight-training routine, 3 times per week (2–3 sets per muscle group)
- Stretching exercises for each major muscle groups

Mostly Cardio Talk

Once you've entered the world of the Busy Mom's Advanced Exercise Plan, you pretty much plan on knocking out at least 20 minutes of cardio work at a pop. Other times, you get in a longer workout. It could be 30 minutes, maybe 45, or even an hour occasionally. A full hour, you say? While that concept may sound foreign to some busy moms, once you're at the advanced level, it's certainly a possibility, at least on occasion. Varying the amount of time you spend on your aerobic workout keeps the body guessing. It also allows you to vary the intensity of your workouts. You've got only 20 minutes? Shoot for higher intensity or intervals. Got some extra time? Take it down a notch and just keep going. (I still like to sprinkle some high intensity intervals in here, too!) Varying the type of aerobic activity is a great idea also. We covered this in the chapter on aerobic exercise. It's never the best idea to stress the same muscles and the same joints in the same way every day. It can lead to injury and also lessen the results. After all, the body has no need to adapt when it can predict your every move.

My own workout habits are a good example of varying the type, intensity, and length of cardio workouts based on the day at hand. Mondays are currently my day to sleep in (if you can call it that!). I don't work out in the early morning because I teach a mid-morning interval step aerobics class that day. It's a lot of fun and a great change of pace from my normal workout that gets in both an aerobic workout and weight training. Then, I have a commitment to myself to work out every Wednesday and Friday in the early morning at home. The "plan" is for me to get up about an hour before the rest of the household and get it done before everyone else needs me. I usually do about 30 minutes on the treadmill or walking/jogging outside, followed by 2–3 sets of weights per body part. Tuesdays and Thursdays are bonus days when I only do cardio, so I have time for more than 30 minutes if I get up on time. I must admit that almost half the time (for instance if I've been up late writing into the wee hours!), I ignore the alarm clock (and my husband kicking me) and wait almost a full hour before finally jumping out of bed and tearing downstairs for a quick 20 minutes on the treadmill, followed by whatever weights I can get done in about 10 minutes if it's a "weights day." I'm left with barely enough time to pack the lunchboxes and get the kids on the school bus while still in my sweaty exercise clothes. Ideal? No. Done? Yes! Busy moms who work outside the home can easily apply my technique to their situation as well. It's all about hedging the clock with the variables at hand and getting in what you can.

Varying the amount of time you spend on your aerobic workout keeps the body guessing.

Another great change of pace is the occasional extra-long aerobic workout. I aim for one 60-minute cardio workout each week, although I admit it doesn't usually happen that often unless it's the warm summer months. In the summer, I love to go for really long, brisk walks with a neighbor or two after the kids have gone to bed. We're so busy chatting that we hardly notice that an hour's gone by. And we look forward to our walks so much that we often go three or more nights a week. In the winter, the best I can do is the occasional weekend day when there is something really good on TV that can pass the time on the treadmill for that long. Gym-goers might get in a 60-minute cardio without boredom by varying the type, like doing 20 minutes each on the treadmill, elliptical, and stair climber. Remember that it's only once you're mentally and logistically ready for the advanced level, that you can take heed of the fact that long cardio workouts (i.e. 45–60 minutes) are the ticket to weight loss. The quickie cardios aren't going to help you as much in that area, but I hate to put too much emphasis on that for the sake of our beginner and intermediate friends. Those busy moms are still doing great things for themselves and just need a little more time (for the weight to come off and/or for them to feel ready to graduate to the advanced level), and a lot more patience and acceptance. Remember, they should be patting themselves on the back that they are doing it *at all!* The good news is that week in and week out, it doesn't really matter how long your aerobic workout is. Get in what you can get in and then move on with your day. Remember my motto, "More may be better than less, but some is better than none."

More on Weights

The advanced level weight-training routine is G-R-E-A-T! At this point, you really start understanding which exercises match each muscle group, and you probably have more than one exercise per muscle group in your bag of tricks. However, you're still part of the advanced club if you simply have one exercise per muscle group and do two sets of each. It's more than the intermediate level and the added stimulus will increase the tone and strength gains you receive. The "three sets per muscle group" routine is regulation-issue core recommendations for awesome benefits without crossing over to the world of people who have hours to spend in the gym. (Those types may do two or even three exercises per body part and do three sets of each exercise. That's a total of six to nine sets per muscle group!) I don't know many busy moms who have time for that! Three sets per muscle group is definitely a workable routine, at least some of the time. And again, once you're in the advanced mindset, you probably can make it work if you want to. The reason it's great? I believe there is simply some manner of physiological threshold about three sets. When you start doing three sets per muscle group, you'll likely see an exponential increase in the gains you make in strength, firmness, and definition of your muscles. It's best not to lock yourself in to only one exercise per body part. Three sets gives you the opportunity to mix and match which exercises you'll do each day. For instance, the bench press, dumbbell flies, and push-ups all work the chest muscles. One day, you may decide to do three sets of bench press. Another day, two sets of bench press and one set of dumbbell flies. The third day, you might do one set each of bench press, dumbbell flies, and push-ups. Each exercise works the chest muscles in a slightly different way and that is good!

And don't forget — just because you try to do three sets per muscle group on most days, that doesn't mean you can't have a day when you just do two or even one set per muscle group if that's all that will work into your schedule. Congratulate yourself on giving your muscles some stimulation and check it off your list as done!

The Busy Mom's Advanced Weight Training Routine

Okay, so you're doing two or three sets per muscle group, and you want to have several exercises you can choose from for each muscle group. If you're working out at a gym, take a look at the weight training equipment that is set up like stations. Most likely, each piece of equipment has a helpful little card that shows the name of the muscle it works, usually with a picture. It will also describe how to correctly perform the exercise. The only problem is that many busy moms don't know how each exercise fits into the big picture. Using the list on the next few pages as a guide, you will know which muscle groups you need to hit (there are 11 total), as well as several options for each. This list of exercises (and muscle groups, for that matter) is by no means definitive. There are some smaller muscle groups that hard-core fitness enthusiasts like to work in a more specialized way. We won't go there in this book. And, there are many different exercises and machines for each major muscle group, whether you are working out at home or at a gym. We'll concentrate on the exercises you'd do at home, because if you're going to a gym, chances are the staff can help you with the available equipment at their facility.

Let's take a look at a few of the more common exercises for each muscle group. Don't forget that some exercises hit more than one muscle group. Those kinds of exercises, such as squats and lunges, are the best way to get the most bang for your buck! Pictures and details on how to perform each exercise are beyond the scope of this book. Fledgling advanced-level moms can stick to the exercises pictured in the Busy Mom's Intermediate Exercise Plan — but at an advanced intensity (basically 2–3 sets instead of one). If you are a more seasoned advanced mom, you will see a few on this list that you are familiar with and have access to. Go for it!

You can also check out www.busymomsolutions.com for more resources in this area.

The Busy Mom's Advanced Weight Training Exercises

Choose from the Following Exercises to Target Each Muscle Group

You don't need to do all of them, but it is a good idea to vary your choices.

Shoulders

- Overhead press (dumbbells)
- Side raise (dumbbells)
- Front raise (dumbbells)
- Rear raise (dumbbells)
- Upright Row (dumbbells or bar)
- Lateral raise machine
- Military Press machine

Chest

- Chest press (bar, dumbbells, or machine)
- Dumbbell flies
- Push-ups
- Cable cross-overs

Back

- Lat pull machine — close grip
- Lat pull machine — wide grip
- Seated Row — machine
- Tubing row
- T-bar row (in the free weights section of the gym)

The Busy Mom's Advanced Weight Training Exercises (cont'd)

Biceps (front of the arm)

- Dumbbell curls
- Concentration curls
- Bicep curl machine
- Bicep curls with tubing

Triceps (back of the arm)

- Dumbbell overhead extension
- Tricep pushdown (bar or rope)
- Overhead tricep extension with rope (on lat pull machine)
- Tricep extension with tubing (overhead or off to the side)
- Dumbbell tricep kickback
- Modified dips

Abdominals (stomach area)

- Crunches (fast, slow, hold up for three counts and then lower down for one count, etc.)
- Reverse curls (lifting the hips off of the floor)

Quadriceps (front of the thigh)

- Squats (bar, dumbbell, ball)
- Lunges (walking, stationary, with or without dumbbells)
- Leg Press machine
- Squat machine
- Leg Extension machine

The Busy Mom's Advanced Weight Training Exercises (cont'd)

Hamstrings (back of the thigh)

- Hamstring curl machine
- Ball hamstring curl

Gluteus Maximus (rear end)

- Squats (bar, dumbbell, ball)
- Lunges (walking, stationary, with or without dumbbells)
- Hip extensions on knees and forearms
- Glute isolation machine

Hips (note that your hip muscles are not on your outer thigh, they are above your hip joint)

- Hip abduction using tubing with handles, lying down
- Hip abduction using tubing rings, standing
- Side-lying hip abduction
- Hip abduction machine

Inner Thigh

- Ball squeezes
- Inner thigh machine

How to Get Done Quickly with Multiple Sets Per Muscle Group

When you are doing more than one set per muscle group, your body needs to have between 30 seconds and 2 minutes rest between sets. This is called your recovery time. If you try to do another set for the same muscle group without a little rest, you'll soon find out that you won't get very far! The heavier the weight/fewer the reps, the longer the rest interval needed, but it's pretty subjective. Some gym-goers with lots of time on their hands do one set of bench press, for example, stand around chit-chatting for a few minutes waiting for their muscles to recover, and then do their next set of bench press. This is not the way of the busy mom. The busy mom will want to make the best use of her time whether she's working out at home or at a gym. There are several ways to do this. First of all, remember the rule about always working your chest and back *before* you work your biceps and triceps, unless you want wet noodles for arms with which to perform your back and chest exercises. Then, you sequence your exercises so that while one muscle group is resting in between sets, you are using that time to work a different muscle group. Circuit training is one method that many people use in which they do one set for every muscle group and then start again from the beginning for their second and/or third set. This is a fine way to work out, but it isn't my favorite, because each muscle group is getting quite a long rest between sets. I prefer to completely focus on and fatigue a muscle group and then move on. The method I recommend for alternating exercises has two ways you could do it: alternate opposing muscle groups (chest-back-chest-back) or alternate upper and lower body muscle groups (chest-hamstrings-chest-hamstrings). Both systems have their merit. Alternating upper and lower body exercises allows the muscles to really recover because you are not working anywhere near where you just were. Alternating opposing muscle groups might be good on a day when you want to work a little harder. Technically, the just-worked muscle is taking a break while you work the opposite muscle group, but it is still called upon a bit for stabilization.

Here's my favorite routine:

1. Alternate Bench Press (chest) and Hamstring Curls for 2 or 3 sets each
2. Alternate Lat Pull (back) and Side Raises (shoulders) for 2 or 3 sets each
3. Rotate through Squats (glutes and quads), Bicep Curls, and Triceps Pushdowns for 2 or 3 sets each
4. Alternate Inner Thigh Ball Squeeze and Hip Abduction for 2 or 3 sets each
5. Abdominal Crunches

When I do this routine, I can fly through it and it just feels good to me. Don't forget that it's a good idea to vary the sequencing every now and then. Try different sequences based on the layout of your equipment and personal preferences. Think about efficiency of time and plan out your routine so that you minimize time wasters like getting up and down off of the floor repeatedly, or having to change equipment settings. While you are actually doing the exercises, though, that's not the time to rush! Keep your movements steady and controlled.

The Busy Mom's Advanced Exercise Plan Stretching Routine

After a Cardio Workout

Be sure to stretch your calves, quadriceps, and hamstrings, referring to the stretches for these muscle groups listed in Appendix 2.

After Working Your Abdominal Muscles

Stretch your abdominal muscles by reaching your arms overhead while lying on the floor. Be sure to stretch your lower back muscles by pulling your knees into your chest.

During Your Weight Training Routine

When you are lifting weights at an advanced level, it's a great idea to stretch each muscle group right after you work it. Refer to the stretches listed in Appendix 2. It only takes a few seconds and feels really good. Hold each position for 10-30 seconds before moving to your next weight training exercise.

The Benefits

We've reached the highest point in our cumulative list of the benefits of exercise as we've worked through the levels. The benefits of the Busy Mom's Advanced Exercise Plan are incredible! You have really arrived. Here they are:

✔ All of the benefits listed in the Busy Mom's "I'm Not Going to Change into Exercise Clothes" Plan, as well as those listed in the Busy Mom's Beginner Exercise and Intermediate Exercise Plans **but to an exponentially larger degree!** You are doing so much more exercise and at increased intensities that you'll find noticeable differences!

- ❖ Improved general health.
- ❖ Increased energy.
- ❖ Reduced risk of a host of chronic diseases — heart disease, diabetes, and some cancers.
- ❖ Consistency with an intentional effort toward fitness.
- ❖ A fitness-conscious mindset that may lead to a lifetime of exercise!
- ❖ Improved strength and capacity of your heart and lungs.
- ❖ Improved blood pressure.
- ❖ Increased muscular endurance and tone in many muscle groups from the aerobic activity.

- ❖ An outlet for stress.
- ❖ Improved sleep patterns.
- ❖ Stronger and more taut abdominal muscles leading to improved appearance.
- ❖ Alleviation or prevention of lower back pain.
- ❖ A sense of accomplishment and possibly a hankering for more exercise down the road.

Plus:

- ✔ Even greater increases in muscular strength and endurance for all of your major muscles groups.
- ✔ An even greater increase in metabolic rate and calorie burning.
- ✔ Even greater improvement in aerobic capacity/cardiovascular endurance.
- ✔ Help with weight loss due to more substantial increases in metabolism and calorie burning.

What's Next?

Once you are living the flexible advanced exercise level lifestyle, enjoy it and see where it takes you. You may be content to keep your routine pretty consistent, just like many of us are content to eat the same thing for breakfast or lunch every day. Others crave variety and feel the need to change things more often. For instance, after having a certain pattern for three or six months, you may find yourself getting bored. If that's you, start sniffing around for ways to change things up. Your ears might perk up about an upcoming long-distance walk for charity. Training for that walk becomes your focal point, you'll meet new people, and have a fabulous sense of accomplishment. Or, you may decide to hire a personal trainer for a few sessions to pick up some new exercise ideas. Or, you may check out the local gym and start mixing some exercise classes into your usually solo exercise habits. Or, you decide it's finally time to invest in a little more substantial home exercise equipment. There are tons of ideas for the taking! Go for it!

• SECTION FOUR •
A Busy Mom's Call to Action

Chapter 15

Location, Location, Location

The Busy Mom's Exercise Levels focus on choices about how much or how little you do. Now it's time to focus on *where and when* you will exercise. I'm sure you've heard the mantra about the most important factor in buying a home — location, location, location. Well, this mantra also holds true for the busy mom's exercise efforts. Obviously, there are many places that you can exercise, and we'll talk about some of the more common options. Most consistent exercisers have a plan that includes *more than one location.* It's all about having a back-up plan, right?

Home Exercise

As you can tell from the routines I created in this book, I'm a big fan of home exercise for busy moms. You always have everything with you and you don't need to leave the house. You can't beat the convenience and the flexibility of a home exercise program if you have the discipline to really do it. You can work out at any time, day or night, with the kids around or without. You can easily implement the beginner, intermediate, or even advanced exercise plans at home. If you want an even more personalized home workout, don't rule out hiring a personal trainer for at least a few sessions to get you going. You can then schedule an appointment every now and then to upgrade your program and keep you motivated. You can do a full routine with minimal equipment, or you can gradually invest in some of the more expensive home equipment when you are sure you'll use it.

Home Exercise Equipment

In the intermediate exercise plan, I introduced you to a complete home exercise program you could do with just a few dumbbells, exercise tubing, and a large, inflatable exercise ball. Once you are on a roll, investing in a piece of aerobic equipment is a great addition for those winter months when it's too cold to walk outside. Or, advanced level busy moms might want to invest in a multi-station weight-training setup that allows you to do more advanced weight-training exercises. When purchasing exercise equipment, make sure you go to a reputable exercise equipment store where the sales staff can answer questions and where you can actually try out the equipment. Similar pieces of equipment from different manufacturers vary in how they feel and operate. If you go shopping for a treadmill, for example, go in your exercise clothes and try several different models. You will find one that has the best feel for you. You'll also be looking for value and quality. Don't be in a hurry to buy. There will always be another sale. Make sure you've done your homework before purchasing.

Videotapes or DVDs

For some busy moms, exercise videotapes or DVDs can be a great alternative. You've got someone showing you exactly how to do each exercise, in the privacy of your own home, anytime you want to do it! The videos can get boring after a while though, if you don't keep a variety on hand. I know busy moms who collect exercise videos like shoes. They have a whole collection and when it's time to exercise, they see what they are in the mood for. You can find exercise videos for your aerobic workout, weight training, stretching, as well as many specialty workouts. Another great feature of some videos is that they are often broken up into sections, so you can do little mini workouts if that's all you have time for. Be sure to look for videos or DVDs that feature credentialed fitness experts, not just celebrities. One great resource is www.collagevideo.com. They have a huge selection of quality exercise videos with detailed descriptions and ratings of each video, and customer service agents who actually use the exercise videos in order to give a first hand opinion when possible.

Full Service Health Clubs

A full-service health club can be a great option for many busy moms. With a variety of cardio equipment, weights, and classes to choose from, your fitness needs can certainly be met. Here's what to look for in a full-service health club:

- Convenience – Is the location convenient to your home or work (whichever place you'll be coming from) and are the hours sufficient for when you'll want to work out?
- A warm and inviting atmosphere – You will get a vibe the minute you walk in the door. Is it a good vibe?
- A free trial – Whether it's one day or one week, most clubs should offer a chance to test out the club to see if you like it. Make sure you visit the club at the time you plan to exercise so that you can see how crowded it is.
- Additional amenities – Are you interested in a pool or posh locker room area?
- Class schedule – If you are interested in group exercise classes, such as step aerobics, spinning, or yoga, make sure the schedule meets your interests and times you are available to come.
- A knowledgeable, friendly and helpful staff – Are there certified trainers there to show you what to do and take an interest in getting to know you?

- Child Care — The better clubs will have on-site child care. Check it out to see if you get a good feeling. Talk to other moms who use it.
- Look for clubs that charge monthly fees, rather than those that push long-term, pay-ahead contracts. If they already have your money, what's their incentive to keep you happy? And if you don't actually use the club regularly, even better for them. It'll make the club less crowded for future prospects.

Women-only Quick Workout Centers

No-frills, inexpensive, women-only clubs are popping up all over the country, and with good reason. These fitness clubs, such as Curves,™ are attracting women in droves with their promise of a full workout in less than 30 minutes in an atmosphere that is casual and supportive. Interestingly enough, statistics show that the popularity of these types of clubs is not taking members away from full-service health clubs. Rather, these types of clubs are reaching women who wouldn't set foot in a traditional health club because they live in a rural setting with none nearby, or because the clubs are too expensive or intimidating. The equipment is minimal and many are organized into a circuit of weight training machines alternated with mini-trampolines for alternating cardio with resistance training. A busy mom who fits into the "I'm not going to change into exercise clothes", beginner, or intermediate levels might be a good candidate for this setting. Any busy mom used to a strenuous or advanced exercise routine will find these workouts not quite challenging enough. The drawbacks include the Spartan surroundings and the lack of childcare and other amenities. But, their philosophy is bare bones for an affordable price and it's working for many women.

Community Centers and County Recreation Facilities

You may be surprised what's available once you start looking. Often, there are exercise facilities in community centers and county recreation facilities that are well equipped, albeit without any special amenities, and usually have much lower membership fees, and are less crowded than health clubs. What about those County Recreation classes? You might be able to find exercise classes happening in the evenings at a public elementary school near you. They often run in cycles, such as 12 weeks. If this appeals to you, it's an internet search away!

Lynn works in a busy office and has a family to care for at home. When she first meets with me, she says that she doesn't want to feel so tired all the time or look frumpy beyond her years. She wants to put a spring back in her step and look a little trimmer, maybe buy some new clothes to feel good in. So we start talking about how the pieces to the puzzle could fit together for her. She decides that exercising in the morning before work is the only time that's going to fit her schedule. Now, morning is not for everyone — especially for a new habit. Lynn promises me she's not one to hit the snooze button a dozen times so we give it a shot. The community center near her home has a well-equipped fitness room for a very reasonable monthly fee. We meet there 3 or 4 times to set up an exercise routine that will take her no more than 45 minutes three times a week. We decide to start small with the eating changes. We set some basic guidelines for good food choices and detail a handful of weekly goals. Week by week, steady as she goes, Lynn begins to make progress and get excited. She emails me that after doing the treadmill, she thought it would be fun to add 15 minutes on the elliptical trainer as well, and asks if that's ok. Well . . . YES! Next, it's about the weights. She's anxious to add a second set of each exercise, and maybe one extra cardio workout on the weekends. Her family is starting to get used to the fact that she's buying whole wheat bread and skim milk. She's even starting to collect healthy dinner recipes and reports that the food critics at home have given most of them a thumb's up! Lynn and I talk on the phone every three weeks to check in and set new weekly goals. She has lost almost ten pounds, but more importantly to her, she exudes excitement. She says it feels like a cloud has been lifted and everything looks different now.

Support Is Available If You Need It

Well, I have to admit that I'm biased. Since I am both a personal trainer and a fitness and wellness coach, of course I believe in the value! I have written this book as both a trainer and a coach so you are already well on your way. By reading this far, you should be aware of the kind of information and support that is available from these types of fitness professionals. Imagine how much more support you could receive from someone focusing specifically on you, your goals, and your situation. Let me first say that these options are not just for the moms with money. You'd be surprised at how affordable it can be when you space out how and when you use a trainer or coach. For some families, it certainly may be completely out of the question financially. But for others, let's be honest about how we spend our discretionary income. If you've tried and failed multiple times before without support, isn't it worth considering? After all, our theme throughout this book is, "What's going to make this time different?"

Personal Trainers

We spent some time in Section One covering fitness and wellness coaches. Let's take a closer look at what a personal trainer has to offer. A personal trainer will design an exercise program specifically for you based on your special needs and preferences. This could be an invaluable service if you have specific problems like old injuries or joint problems. A trainer could also be a source of structure and accountability. After all, it's hard to blow off a workout when you have an appointment to keep with someone. Your trainer will also provide support and motivation. You'll likely work harder with your trainer and enjoy doing so! Your trainer can provide the continuity to your exercise efforts and some much needed pampering. I have many busy mom clients who tell me that their workouts with me are their respite away from their daily grind with the kids and/or their job. Your trainer will give you piece of mind that you are doing each exercise correctly so that you don't injure yourself. With your trainer, you'll be able to track your progress toward your goals on an on-going basis, and change your workouts along the way so that you are always getting the best workout to meet your goals. Personal trainers can be used as often or as seldom as you'd like. Once you have someone with whom you feel a rapport, how often you schedule appointments is mostly a question of budget. I have many clients who do the majority of their workouts on their own, but work with me for their one or two "hard" workouts each week. These are the days they plan to really push themselves and work with equipment they don't have access to on their own. They do additional workouts at home, or they even belong to a club to use other days of the week. If it sounds appealing to you, why not do a little research?

What to Look for in a Personal Trainer

It's a good idea when considering hiring a personal trainer to interview several before making any decisions. You'll want to compare their credentials, experience, and the rapport that you feel with them. The importance of rapport shouldn't be underestimated. You should feel a personal connection with your trainer because you will be spending a lot of time with them. Never hire a trainer with whom you feel awkward around or who doesn't seem to be genuinely interested in you, regardless of their credentials. I'd look for a trainer who has a degree in exercise science in addition to a certification or two from a nationally recognized organization such as ACSM, ACE, or NSCA. (You can check out the websites for these three organizations in the References section.) You'll also want to look for a trainer who has at least several years of experience working with clients who have needs similar to yours.

How about a Fitness Friend?

Personal trainers and coaches aren't the only way to get outside support for your fitness efforts. Finding a friend who you can exercise with (or at least check in with) can also help you stick with your exercise program when the going gets tough. It will be more fun than exercising alone and it will be harder to cancel if someone else is expecting you.

Remember, location and support are two of the most important factors to consider so that you can be successful with your exercise efforts!

Chapter 16

Real World Tips for Stay-at-home Moms and Work-outside-of-the-home Moms

First and foremost, we all know that whether you work outside of the home or inside of the home, if you're a mom, you are working – period! That being said, I purposely didn't make a huge issue about being a stay-at-home mom vs. a work-outside-of-the-home mom in this book. Rather than focus on the differences that sometimes cause tension between working and stay-at-home moms (working moms feeling judged for leaving their children, stay-at-home moms feeling judged that they abandoned their career ambitions), there is much we can do to support each other. While each of these two groups have unique challenges and unique opportunities, they are more similar than dissimilar, not to mention the existence of a whole lot of in-between moms (like me!). Sure, the media would have you believe that you're either a "working mom" or a "stay-at-home mom", but truth be told, there seems to be as many arrangements out there as there are moms! We are indeed rewriting the rulebooks and creating situations that work for our unique family and career situations. We can recognize that each mom has made a very personal decision based on her unique situation. I believe that every mom's decision to work outside of the home or not is based on how a number of factors uniquely blend together for her situation.

So, let's get to discussing a few of the unique challenges and tips for stay-at-home moms and work-outside-of-the-home moms.

Special Challenges and Solutions for Stay-at-home Moms

Stay-at-home moms definitely have special challenges, starting with the hours, right? You're on duty twenty-four hours a day, seven days a week. You may be strapped financially because you stopped working, exhausted from bickering kids and a messy house, and frustrated because you don't have childcare to do those things that working moms may take for granted – a nice lunch out at a restaurant every now and then or a chance to run errands or even get a haircut without an entourage. You may be home all day, but you're certainly not watching TV and eating chocolates! Have you heard the joke about the husband who comes home one day to find the house an absolute disaster, with trash and dishes everywhere and kids running amok while the wife was sitting on the couch with a magazine? The husband asks, "What's going on here?" The wife answers, "Well honey, every day when you come home and see the house looking exactly as it did when you left, you ask me what I did that day. Well, today I didn't do it!"

There are more tips coming in the *Special Tips for Stages with the Ages* section, but first let's look at some ideas for stay-at-home moms. Of course, not all of the tips will apply to you. For instance, you might have a husband who works a ton of hours or travels a lot, but there still has to be a way to fit a little bit of activity into your day if you really want to.

- When you are straightening up the house or doing laundry, don't build a pile at the bottom of the stairs to bring upstairs later. Go ahead and make those trips up and down the stairs as needed.

- Get in the habit of walking to the bus stop, or to the playground, or wherever. There are probably places you could walk to instead of driving. Start noticing how quickly you decide to hop in the car.
- Back to the bus stop — how about wearing exercise clothes to the bus stop and starting your walk right after you finish waving goodbye? You'll get a workout in before you set foot back in the house.
- Get some exercise yourself when you take your children to sports practice. Are there times when you stay at a particular practice because it doesn't make sense to go home and come back? When I take my daughter to soccer practice, I may wear exercise clothes and take a walk around the soccer fields with a few of the other moms while the kids are practicing.
- Build activity into playgroups. In the warm weather, meet for stroller walks with your other mom friends instead of sitting around the kitchen table while the kids play.
- Join a health club that has childcare. You'll probably find exercise classes in the mid-morning filled with other moms just like you. Feeling part of a group and having a network of fitness-oriented mom friends will make a difference in your efforts.
- If you're part of a two-parent household, get up early one or two mornings a week and get a workout in before your husband or significant other leaves for work. Let them handle breakfast and the rest of the kids' morning routine. After all, you're on duty for the rest of the day after they leave. It's the least they can do, right? Or get up even earlier. There's something very satisfying about having already logged a workout and showering for the day before anyone else is up. Not every day, mind you! But give it a try. You may only have to get up a little earlier than usual.
- Have a serious heart-to-heart talk with your husband or other family member or support person about how

you can make this work, given that exercise is important to you. Maybe you can get them to agree to come home early one or two nights a week so that you can get out of the house and get to the gym.

- Stake a claim on some weekend time to exercise, since you're on duty Monday through Friday. Get family members used to a routine where you get 45 minutes to exercise every Saturday.
- In the summer months, walk with a few neighbors after the kids are in bed. (This is my favorite!)
- Train your mind that the laundry and the dishes and the stack of paper on the kitchen counter really can wait. I live the life. I know there is a lot to do around the house. You don't have to pick exercise every time, but you do have to pick it some of the time. Feel good that you are doing something for yourself. You deserve it!

It isn't easy, but the extra energy you'll gain by getting more active will be well worth it. You can do it!

Special Challenges and Solutions for Work-outside-of-the-home Moms

Challenges? Let's see. How about: not enough time in the day, guilt, stress, being pulled in two different directions, traffic, late fees at childcare, deadlines, a boss who doesn't understand, and a dirty house. You have a sick child or a snow day coinciding with a major presentation at work. You probably don't need me to go on — you're living it. I lived it for several years, too. Are you a working mom who isn't exercising because you feel as though you're already away from your kids too much? Are you wondering how you can justify being away any more than that? I don't have any easy answers. All I can do is refer you back to the benefits that you want . . . that you need from exercise, and remind you that there are shades of gray. You are managing many things in your life and you can manage this, too.

Let's get to solutions. Again, I've got no magic wand. As much as I'd like to, I can't create more hours in the day for you. The question remains, "How are you using the 24 hours in your day?" There *are* working moms who are exercising regularly. Can you be one of them? Don't forget all we've learned so far about "all-or-none" attitudes. I'm not asking you to fit the advanced exercise plan into your life if it's not meant to be right now. Are there some small changes you can make that will be meaningful? Here are some ideas to think about:

- Commit to taking the stairs at work and parking at the far end of the parking lot on a daily basis. (Don't just think it's a great idea . . . make it part of who you are.)
- Don't abuse e-mail. If you have something to tell someone at your workplace, get up out of your chair and go on down the hall to talk to them.
- Hold walking meetings. Of course this won't work for all meetings, but there are bound to be times when you could go for a walk with a co-worker when you need to discuss a project.
- If you're part of a two-parent household, negotiate with your husband or significant other about when you can work out. Make it a serious heat-to-heart, "Honey, this is important to me. How can we make this work?" Then the negotiations begin. "If you handle the kids on Monday and Wednesday mornings while I go in early to workout, I'll do all the other mornings." Grab a weekend workout on top of that and you're in business! Of course, this is just an example. Get a conversation going from a problem-solving perspective and see where it takes you.
- If you are a single parent, figure out when you can exercise within the time you are already away from your kids, or see if there is any flexibility in the drop-off/pick-up times to allow for a super-quick workout one or two days a week.

- Exercise on your lunch hour. Yes, I know this is also the only time you may have to run errands, but you've turned a corner, right? If exercise has moved up on the priority list, then you can take the step of allocating at least a few days per week to moving your body during your lunch hour, right? If there are no facilities to change your clothes, no problem. How about keeping some sneakers at your desk and going for a quick walk?
- Even better, recruit others at work to form a walking group, an exercise support network, or healthy habit buddy system.
- If the weather isn't cooperative for walking outdoors, how about walking inside? Some workplaces are large enough for a good walk inside. You can even be sneaky about it, if need be. Grab a few file folders, walk all the way down the hall, up the stairs, all the way down that hall, up the stairs again, and so on. (Everyone will think you are on your way to an important meeting!)
- Some lucky working moms may have access to a corporate fitness center at their worksite or corporate membership rates at a nearby health club. Use them! Maybe your job is flexible, allowing you to get away from your desk during the day for a quick workout. Or, how about early morning? Once you get used to the "packing your clothes the night before routine," early morning club-goers beat the rush, miss traffic, and still make it to work on time.
- Put your exercise sessions on your calendar just like any other appointment. Your co-workers will get used to it. You wouldn't cancel an appointment with someone else very easily, would you? Why are we so quick to cancel appointments with ourselves?
- Along the same lines, do your part to set the tone at work to value fitness and a balanced lifestyle. Even if you're not the boss, you have a sphere of influence at work. Who knows, maybe you're healthy habits and attitudes will rub off on your co-workers!

- Take a good look at the things that take up your time and energy. It's always good to periodically re-evaluate, especially if you have a tendency to assume the role of super mom. If your commitment to exercise is on the rise, what else can you cut out? You're probably already an expert at consolidating errands and getting the most out of your time, but maybe you can drop a volunteer committee or hire someone to clean the house occasionally. There have to be a few things you can clear from your plate to make room for exercise.
- If you're a morning person, get your workout out of the way at home in the early A.M. If you're starting at the beginner level, we're only talking about getting up 20 minutes early a few days of the week, right?
- What about after work, on your way home? If you can swing the logistics (heart-to-heart talk with your hubby or support person again), go for it! But with dinner to do, homework and baths, and the exhaustion factor, after work doesn't seem to be the best bet for most working moms.
- After the kids go to bed? Again, we're talking about the exhaustion factor. You know yourself best. If you allow yourself the indulgence of watching a TV show or two after the kids have gone to bed, how about walking on the treadmill while watching?

You've got a lot on your plate, but even more at stake if you don't do something to get yourself more active. Pick something and get to it!

A Special Note to Single Moms

When it comes to busy moms, single moms are first on the list. If you are a single mom, your day is longer, your challenges are greater, and your spare time is probably non-existent. When all is said and done, you are the one holding the bag for just about everything where the children and household are concerned. From doctor's appointments to checking homework, packing lunches to fixing leaky faucets, carpooling to doing dishes, it's all you. On top of all that, you are probably working full time and working hard to make the best home you can for your children. For all of those reasons, you may be thinking,

> *"How can I possibly exercise when there's no one else besides me to do all this other stuff? And even if I did get everything done, you'd find me collapsed on the couch — not exercising, thank you very much!"*

So where does this leave us? Let's start with some perspective. You wouldn't be reading this book if you didn't value health and fitness on some level and want to become more fit. You know from reading thus far all of the remarkable benefits you have to gain from leading a healthier lifestyle. And you know that *you alone are the single most important element in the life of your children.* You know intuitively, that you owe it to your kids to take good care of yourself. No one knows better than you that there is so much depending upon you being around and being healthy enough and energetic enough to meet your kids' ongoing needs. But still, there is the issue of time. This is where you take to heart the primary messages of this book (priority and habit) and review the Busy Mom's Exercise Levels in light of your situation. How about:

- Taking a look at your unique motivators and obstacles, and decide what Busy Mom Exercise Level is right for you in this stage of your life. If nothing else, maybe you adopt the "I'm not going to change into exercise clothes" plan or the beginner exercise plan and celebrate it! Maybe it will grow into more as your life changes.
- Seek support from neighbors and friends.
- Exercise with your kids — taking the little ones in the stroller, riding bikes with bigger kids, or playing games outside.

- Use exercise as a small amount of time you take for yourself.
- Commit to little snippets of exercise throughout the day that will add up.

Above all, get in touch with the reasons why this is important to you and believe in yourself that you can make it work. You know that you can! Don't be too hard on yourself and don't set your expectations too high, but do what you can. You are already an expert at juggling. I don't need to tell you how or what to juggle beyond the information in this book that applies to all busy moms. You are the best expert on your life and what will work. Sit down with a paper and pencil, brainstorm some ideas, seek out some support, and commit to something. You can do it!

Special Tips for Stages with the Ages

All of the Busy Mom Exercise Levels discussed in Section Three were designed to have applications for whatever stage of motherhood you are in. But, let's look at a few of the unique opportunities and challenges that come with the ages of your children.

Moms with Infants

Exercise may not be the first thing on your priority list when you are bleary-eyed and sleep deprived. Because of the constant physical demands of having an infant and sheer exhaustion, many busy new moms put exercise on hold. But, you know that I'm going to say that the same two rules apply to the new busy mom:

1. Don't worry about content. Just do what you can as opposed to just scrapping the whole idea all together.
2. Exercise in any amount will **give** you more energy that you so desperately need.

So won't you try? Here are some suggestions:

- Check out Appendix 3 in this book for specific advice on postpartum exercise and a plan for progressing back to your normal exercise routine. Believe it or not, there are valuable things you can be doing *from day one* that will take you just two or three minutes a day.
- Use naptime for exercise, but not all of it and not all the time. All the new mom books say to "sleep when the baby sleeps," and that is true to a certain extent. Especially in the early, early days, your body needs the rest to recharge. In the real world, though, most busy moms I know have a to-do list for naptime as long as their arm. There's no way they're sleeping through the only chance they'll get all day to wash their hair, make a few phone calls in peace, or yes, exercise! Maybe you can decide to use naptime on just one or two days per week for a quick workout.
- Make a commitment to pick one or two other times during the week when you will exercise. In addition to one naptime workout per week, maybe you'll commit to one morning per week and one weekend workout.
- Put the baby in the Baby Bjorn® or other front carrier or in the stroller and go for a walk. It doesn't have to be long. The fresh air will feel great!
- Put the baby on the floor with you and do some abdominal crunches, push-ups, or other exercises every now and then.
- Pair certain exercises with other daily or weekly chores so that you remember to do them. For instance, feeding time could be your cue to do some your Kegel exercises (check out the postnatal section of this book if you don't know what they are.)
- Check to see if there are any "Mommy and Me" type exercise classes near you that are designed for new moms to bring baby along.

Moms with Toddlers and Preschoolers

So now your little one is a whirling dervish of constant energy! Busy moms with toddlers and preschoolers may joke that they don't need to exercise . . . they're already constantly running after their children! While this may be true, let's look for extra opportunities to exercise.

- Put them in the stroller and go for a walk. Don't be too quick to say, "It won't work. They'll want out of the stroller." Keep trying. If you make it a routine and dangle something in it for them, you can turn your walks into something they look forward to. Bring a special snack that they can only have during exercise walks or make sure you end up at the playground or some other fun destination. Daily walks with the stroller were always a part of my exercise routine when my kids were that age. For a while, I don't think my toddlers knew you could go to the playground without "going for a walk" first!
- Actually play with them at the playground! Yes, you could sit on the bench while they play, or you can play chase, kick a ball around, or look for ants with them. Get up and move!
- Turn on some music in the house and dance together. Make up funny dances, play follow-the-leader or hide-and-seek. (Perfect for tiring out your little one before naptime!)
- Let them hang out with you while you do your home exercise routine. There is a time and a place to plunk your child down in front of the TV on occasion and this is it! Will it always go smoothly? Of course not. But they'll get used to the routine and you will get the whole workout in at least some of the time!
- Once again, use naptime for exercise at least on occasion. The laundry and the dishes really can wait sometimes. You deserve to do something for yourself with this time every now and then.

Moms with School-age Kids

Things are getting easier in some ways, but more complicated in others. You may feel like you live in your car, chauffeuring the kids from one activity to the next. Doesn't it seem odd that you spend a good deal of time driving your children to all of their sporting activities so that they can be active and healthy, but you forget your own need for exercise? Now is the time to turn that around and set an example that leading an active lifestyle is important for grown-ups too, not just kids. Keep in mind the following mantras:

1) Our family recognizes the values of fitness.
2) The world does not revolve around my kids' needs. I have needs too, and the kids really can entertain themselves for the small amount of time I need for exercise.

Try these tips:

- Make it a habit to plan fun weekend activities that involve movement for the whole family. Why not try ice-skating or snow tubing in the winter, and hiking or bike riding in the warmer months?
- Take a walk together. Kids and parents can exercise together and share some special time together on a walk. It might not be as fast as you'd go on your own, but it'll be good memories. Another option is for the younger ones to ride their bikes or scooters along with you when you walk.
- Get outside and just play! Soccer, tag, and even touch football don't have to be just for the dads!

There are so many possibilities! Yes, we're living in the real world and there are real obligations, real chores, and real stress, but there are also real solutions for busy moms who want to make it work. You can't expect perfect weeks and I'm not asking you to. However, I am challenging you to get "this stuff" on your conscious mind (most of the time) and do "something" toward this area of your life more often than not. There will still be times when you work late, skip your workout and have cereal for dinner. It's okay. It's a journey. My intent here is to motivate you but to also let you off the hook at times, too. Put your thinking cap on about your own life and figure out how you can make it work! I have faith in you!

Chapter 17

The Energy Factor: You Can Conquer Fatigue

It's another chicken-and-the-egg question isn't it? You don't have the energy to work out, yet you know that regular exercise will give you energy! Am I right? We all know the feeling – dragging a bit after lunch, fighting the urge to nod off on the ride home, that overall aura of blah. You are both collapsed on the couch after the kids are tucked in, only to hear one more request from the top of the stairs for a drink of water. You look at each other and the telepathic negotiation begins. One of you finally utters, "Honey, I'll pay you $1,000 if you take this one."

F-A-T-I-G-U-E. How often during the course of a normal day do you hear someone complain about how tired they are? We are all on a quest for more energy, aren't we? And you don't have to look far to find promises, large and small, for magical sources of energy. You've seen them – energy bars, energy shakes, all kinds of pills and potions on the shelves of your local supplement store. Which one is the latest and greatest, guaranteed to boost energy (and drain your pocketbook)?

Here's another perspective. Entertain the notion that how we feel may be in fact due to a combination of many, small, separately less significant factors that we all take for granted. Separately, they are each just one more thing we know we should do better on, but all together, they spell vibrancy . . . or fatigue.

Why not strive to get a handle on these four culprits of fatigue, rather than look for a magic pill?

1. Stress

Stress takes quite a toll on the body, both physically and psychologically. Anyone who's had the experience of a significant stressor knows that it utterly *drains* you. (Think planning a wedding, surviving a family rift, or dealing with the loss of a loved one.) Yet, we don't often realize that daily, run-of-the-mill stress also has an impact. Taking action to manage stress in your daily life should be the first step to boosting your energy quotient.

2. Dehydration

Fluids play a crucial role in almost all body functions, yet many of us go hours without drinking a thing when we're busy. The simple fact is that water is necessary to keep those billions of cells plumped up, humming along, and your energy up. Water is the best source of hydration — free of calories, sugar, and caffeine.

3. Inactivity

Exercise equals energy. Period. There is nothing like moving your muscles to get oxygen into those lungs and coursing through your body. Increased oxygen usage is vibrancy and cell renewal at its best. With exercise, you invigorate your muscles and your brain. Feel-good hormones abound. They don't call it "runner's high" for nothing!

4. Sleep Deprivation

What do you do when you've got a deadline or to-do list that is way too long? Chances are you probably stay up late or get up early to get the job done. We are constantly stealing nighttime hours for daytime activities, and it takes a toll on the body. Research suggests that getting enough sleep is as important to health as regular exercise and eating right. Besides just feeling crummy, lack of sleep can hinder your brain function, immune system, and even weight loss efforts. It's a hard habit to break, but you can do it. Go to bed!

Want more energy? Trust me and go back to basics. Even more to the point, trust your body. You don't need any special pills or potions. It's kind of like the "Everything I Ever Needed to Know, I Learned in Kindergarten" message. Too often, we underestimate the value of these basics, or just neglect them and hope we can fix it with something we can buy over-the-counter. Manage stress, drink plenty of water, get some exercise, and get some sleep! It's nothing your mother hasn't already told you. It's not glamorous, but it works!

Chapter 18

A Last Word about Motivation

As we start tying all the loose ends together, there is still the nagging awareness that many home treadmills serve as glorified clothing racks, dumbbells lie forgotten under the bed, and gym memberships go unused. The challenge, as we have learned, is accountability. It will always be up to *you*. Nobody can do it *for* you and nobody can take it *from* you. Let's recap some of the more important thoughts on this elusive thing called "motivation."

Keep in Mind . . .

! Exercise is important, but each individual exercise session will never be urgent. For it to work, it must become a priority that you schedule, protect and treat as part of your day. Put it on your calendar like any other appointment and don't be too quick to give it up when something else comes up or someone else demands that their agenda take top priority.

- ! Our fast-paced world is not going to cooperate in helping us find time to be more active. If it's going to happen, it's something you have to take ownership of and work at. The rest of the world is more than happy to keep heaping on the responsibilities until you say "enough."

- ! Avoid all-or-none thinking; this includes categorizing yourself as an "exerciser" or "non-exerciser." More is better than less, but some is better than none. And some will keep the habit in place.

- ! Habit is liquid gold. Treat it as such.

- ! Feel good that you are doing something for yourself and making an investment in your health.

- ! Avoid making short-term goals that may leave you discouraged if you fail.

- ! Exercise is one thing we cannot delegate. Whether you are the president of a corporation or a single mom working two jobs, no*body* can exercise for you but you.

- ! When we are really honest with ourselves, we make time for the things we want to do. Period.

- ! Free yourself from counter-productive thinking, such as comparing yourself to others.

- ! The next year is going to come faster than you think. Do you really want to start and stop an overly-stringent program a dozen times or gradually add some realistic changes to your life that you can maintain for the long haul?

What All Successful Long-Term Exercisers Have in Common

"What do they have that I don't have?" There are busy moms making it work. You may still be struggling to find your fitness solution. You may still be waiting for the click that turns on your internal motivation to exercise regularly. If you want to be successful, model your efforts after those who are being successful, right? What do they have in common?

SOMETHING that acts as a common thread to string the weeks and months together.

When a new routine is young and fragile, you'll need to find some "thing" to serve as a common thread through the weeks and months. It could be a class, an exercise buddy, a personal trainer, or a coach, for example. It doesn't matter what it is that ties the weeks together, but going it alone usually doesn't cut it.

An activity they enjoy.

Taking a walk can be blissful alone time. Taking an exercise class can be great social time. Bike riding with the kids can be great family time. What's going to be fun for you? Whatever it is . . . if it's not fun, no wonder you're not sticking to it.

Flexibility. A back-up plan.

Business travel, a sick child, and deadlines at work can all spell trouble for your exercise consistency unless you've already figured out what you'll do when obstacles arise.

Priority. It's just what they do.

They have the desire to "get a workout in no matter what" on a regular basis. It's not that they never skip a workout, but they feel like something is missing when they do. They get right back on it as soon as they can.

Never fear. If you don't yet have the motivational click, you can get it, all in due time. Surround yourself with the right messages and continue to do your best. Congratulations on what you can do so far! For more tips and reflections from busy moms who are making it work, check out Appendix 4. You may want to refer to it whenever you need some inspiration.

Chapter 19

Get Started!

Today is a Meaningful Part of Your Life
Someday is a dangerous word.
Today is a powerful word.
It is up to *you* to decide how to spend the minutes that make up each day, that make up your life.
It is up to *you* to decide what kind of attitude, attention, and priority to give to all the pieces of your life.
It is up to *you* to decide how you will live every today that makes up your life.

If you need something done, ask a mom. You are your kids' hero. You can do anything. I know you can. You know you can. Can you feel the shift in your attitude and your confidence since Chapter One? You know now that you can and will do something to improve your health and fitness. And you will start today! What's the next step? What have you learned through the pages of this book?

* It all begins with you. Nobody can do this for you.
* There is no magic wand or magic pill.
* Make a commitment to yourself.

* This is an important step in your life. You are determined that *this time will be different* so take the time to take stock and figure out your solution.
* Examine your readiness to change and decide what stage you are in and where you want to be.
* Set realistic, yet tangible, goals.
* Keep your focus on all the benefits you have to gain, especially the ones closest to your heart.
* Anticipate the roadblocks and strategize around them.
* Get a positive mindset and envision success. *Picture* yourself doing it!
* Start slow; just getting there is the goal. The content is less important. Be happy with small steps, heading in the right direction
* Plan it into your day. Wake up thinking about when you're going to be active.
* Seek support. Recruit friends and family members to join you on this journey.
* Find ways to simplify your life and clear out the mental and physical clutter that bogs you down.
* Strive for long-term consistency, not perfection or overnight results.
* You are the best expert on your life. You have to figure out what will work for your life, based on your stage of life and current priorities.
* A healthy lifestyle is a work in progress and a fit lifestyle is progressive.
* It is a journey. There is no finish line.
* Establishing the habit is more important than the content.
* Once the habit is established, the content will probably grow and evolve. *See what happens!*

You may have figured out as you were reading that while the focus of this book was you, the busy mom, the fitness advice and exercise levels can be used by any busy person trying to figure out how they can fit a little fitness into their lives. Be sure to share this information with your friends and family and help inspire them, too, to make fitness a priority in their lives, without it being an all-or-none proposition.

Please let me know how you are doing with *finding your fitness solution!* I care! Visit me at www.busymomsolutions.com. I'll be waiting. When you visit, you will find help, support, and accountability at your fingertips for the asking.

I wish you success, peace of mind, and happiness. I wish good health for you and your families. I wish you laughter and love and tons of fun with your adorable children. They will grow up far too quickly. There's nothing better than being a mom, is there? I'm sure you want to be at your best to care for and enjoy your little ones for many years to come.

My own mother has shown me that being a busy mom doesn't end when your kids grow up. You'll always be a mom, and might just be as busy as ever. Close your eyes and picture the time when *your children* are busy moms and dads themselves. Picture yourself being part of their lives as a strong, healthy, and active grandma. Picture yourself as the "cool grandma" who can do things that all the other grandmas can't do. Finally, picture your adult children who have healthy habits themselves, led by the example of a great mom. Their mom didn't wait to care for her health until she was less busy, for she knew that time would never come. She seized the day and she made it work.

You can do it! What are you waiting for? It's worth it and **you** are worth it!

Appendix 1

Charting Your Course

Remember, the first step for making this time different from all of the other times you've tried to get in shape is taking time to do the mental work before you jump right in to the physical work. You'll have a much clearer idea of where you are going by setting forth a concrete and realistic plan that anticipates the bumps you may encounter along the way. This section is designed to walk you through the motivational and logistical questions you need to ask yourself. You may need to refer back to Chapter 4 as you go through the questions for the background information on each item. Also, these kinds of questions can be difficult to answer if you haven't really thought about them this deeply before. If you'd like to use a wellness or fitness coach to help you work through these questions, contact me at www.fitness-insight.com or contact Wellcoaches ® at www.wellcoaches.com.

Getting Rid of the Baggage

What unhealthy mindsets do you need to get rid of that have undermined your ability to feel good and be successful? (Things like an all-or-none mindset, pessimism, stereotypes, self-consciousness, or an obsession with the quick fix.) List these attitudes and beliefs on the following page.

Where are you in the ***Stages of Change*** for fitness?

- ❒ Precontemplation *(I can't or I won't.)*
- ❒ Contemplation *(I'm thinking about it.)*
- ❒ Preparation *(I'm planning on it.)*
- ❒ Action *(I'm doing it.)*
- ❒ Maintenance *(I'm still doing it.)*

Accepting Ownership and Admitting Priorities

Where do you stand with the mental struggle to accept ownership for making this work? What are you willing to change to put yourself higher up on the priority list?

How will you make time or find time for fitness?

Your Fitness Vision

What does being healthy and fit mean to you? What does it look like? What does it feel like? What do you see in your mind when you picture your "goal self" with regards to health and fitness? Where do you see yourself in one year? Five years? Are there certain things that you are doing regularly, ways you are feeling on a scale of 1–10? When you can visualize what you are trying to attain, it makes it that much easier to get there. Write your fitness vision here:

Your Motivators

Ask yourself: Why do I want this vision? What do I have to gain? Why is this important to me? What is going to be so great when this habit is changed? What would be so bad if I never changed this behavior? Make the list as long as possible and don't hold back. Include the short and silly reasons, as well as the serious and heartfelt. Which items really speak to you and are compelling enough to make you *act?* Put an asterisk next to the most *compelling* motivator(s) on your list.

Your Obstacles

What's going to get in the way? What's too hard about this? Why haven't you succeeded before? You will probably have no problem filling in this list! Some obstacles might be *external* (time constraints, no one to watch the kids), others might be *internal* (an all-or-none attitude, not putting yourself on the priority list). Being specific is important since your next step is problem solving.

Your Strategies for Overcoming Your Obstacles

Most obstacles aren't insurmountable; they just require thoughtful strategizing as well as a commitment to keep plugging away even when things aren't perfect. Try to think of specific strategies to address your obstacles listed previously.

Your Three-month Goals

Three months is far enough away to make substantial change during this time frame, yet close enough to maintain a sense of immediacy and motivation to meet these goals. You may want to make several results-oriented three-month goals (a certain amount of weight lost, being able to walk or jog for a specific amount of time). However, I find three-month goals revolving around habits to be even better (i.e., to be regularly exercising 3 times per week, to be consistently choosing water to drink with meals instead of soda). In this way, you may use each week during the three months to gradually incorporate these habits into your day-to-day routine. Remember, your goals should be S-M-A-R-T (specific, measurable, action-oriented, realistic, and time-sensitive).

____

____

____

____

____

____

____

____

____

____

____

Your First Week's Goals

What small steps can you take this week that will help you begin moving toward your three-month goals?

____

____

____

____

____

Ongoing Weekly Goals

Breaking your three-month goals down into small steps each week can be a very powerful tool to keep you moving forward without overwhelming you. Each week you can assess how you did on your previous week's goals, think about what lessons you learned about yourself, and create another set of goals for the upcoming week. You will probably want to use a notebook or some other tool for writing these weekly goals in one place and recording how well you did and lessons learned. Remember, stringing the weeks together with consistent, focused attention is what leads to success!

Know Thyself — Preferences and Personality

Do you like to have alone time when you exercise or do you crave a fun, social atmosphere? Do you prefer variety and get bored easily or are you most successful when you have a structured, predictable workout that you don't have to think about? When is your energy highest? Are you an early morning person or a night owl? Do you like to chop things up into small, manageable bites or "get it all over with?" Do you get overwhelmed easily or do you prefer to dive into new things? Write it all here!

Find a Common Thread To Stay on Track

Remember, one of the most valuable things that can contribute to your success, especially during the fragile beginning period, is *some kind of common thread that strings the weeks together to become months and then years of a sensible approach and a healthy lifestyle.* It's not good when it's just you against the world! Your common thread helps you stay the course over time. It could be a fitness buddy, a specific class, or a personal trainer, for example. What's going to be your common thread?

Your Busy Mom's Exercise Level Base Style

This is the Busy Mom's Exercise Level that you think best fits your schedule and goals right now.

- ❒ The Busy Mom's "I'm Not Going to Change Into Exercise Clothes" Plan
- ❒ The Busy Mom's Beginner Exercise Plan
- ❒ The Busy Mom's Intermediate Exercise Plan
- ❒ The Busy Mom's Advanced Exercise Plan

Your Toolkit

Which of the following tools will you use to help you stay on track?

- ❒ A Goal-setting Journal
- ❒ Posting or periodically reviewing motivational information (i.e., *64 Reasons to Exercise* and *Words of Wisdom from Busy Moms Who Are Making It Work* from Appendices 4 and 5.)
- ❒ Posting your fitness vision and/or motivators somewhere prominent
- ❒ Pedometer (The ultimate goal is 10,000 steps a day or more. Try to increase your steps by a few hundred per day and build up.)
- ❒ Home Exercise Equipment (dumbbells, tubing and exercise ball)
- ❒ Aerobic exercise equipment for easy home use, especially in the winter (treadmill, elliptical trainer, etc.)
- ❒ Health Club membership
- ❒ Personal Trainer (just for start-up help or ongoing)
- ❒ Fitness or Wellness Coach

Your Checklist for Fitness Plan Success

- ❐ Is it fun?
- ❐ Is it convenient?
- ❐ Is it flexible?
- ❐ Do you have a back-up plan?

  What is it? ______________________________
- ❐ Have you planned it into your day?
- ❐ Have you written your workouts on your calendar just like any other appointment?
- ❐ Do you plan to protect that written appointment unless there is an emergency?

Appendix 2

The Exercises

The Busy Mom's Intermediate Weight Training Routine

There are ten exercises in the Busy Mom's Intermediate Weight Training Routine:

1. **Dumbbell Chest Press (with pushups as an alternate exercise) (chest)**
2. **Seated Tubing Row (back)**
3. **Dumbbell Side Raise (shoulders)**
4. **Dumbbell Bicep Curl (biceps/front of arm)**
5. **Overhead Tricep Extension with a Dumbbell (triceps/back of arm)**
6. **Ball Squat or Dumbbell Squat (quadriceps/front of thigh and gluteus maximus/rear end)**
7. **Ball Hamstring Curl (hamstrings/back of thigh)**
8. **Inner Thigh Ball Squeeze (inner thigh)**
9. **Hip Abduction with Tubing (hips)**
10. **Crunches (abdominal muscles)**

A Note about Sequencing

The ten exercises in the Busy Mom's Intermediate weight training routine are listed with all the upper body exercises together, followed by the lower body exercises, and finally abdominals. This is the most common way to visually organize the list, however, the exercises do not need to be performed in this order. You may find that alternating upper body exercises with lower body exercises prevents undue fatigue concentrated in one area.

Here are the exercises in detail with photos:

1. Dumbbell Chest Press or Pushups (chest)

If you have access to a weight bench or some other place where you can lie on your back and let your arms hang below your body, a dumbbell chest press is your best bet to work your chest muscles. You can also try doing the chest press on the ball as pictured. You'll find that if you try to do them on the floor, you won't be able to get enough range of motion to feel as though you are gaining the benefit. Your alternate exercise is the trusty old push up if you don't have anywhere to do the dumbbell chest press.

Dumbbell Chest Press

If you are using a bench, lie on your back, preferably with your feet up so that your back isn't arched too much. If you are using an exercise ball, sit on it and then walk your feet out until you are lying on the ball as pictured. Extend your arms up directly over your chest, with your elbows mostly straight. Slowly bring your elbows down until the inside end of each dumbbell is touching the outside of your chest/armpit area. Bring the dumbbells back up to the starting position, keeping the dumbbells straight up over your chest (don't let them drift over your face or stomach).

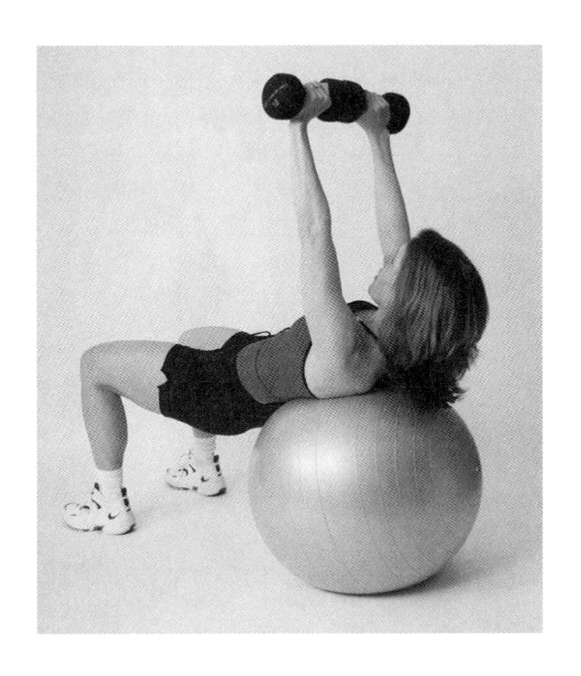

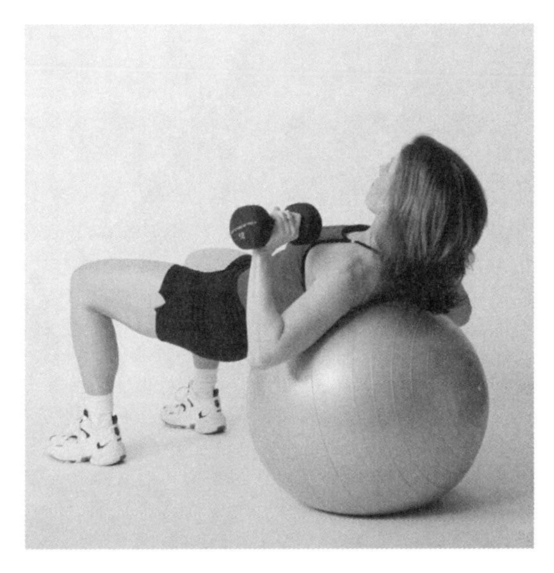

Dumbell Chest Press (start and finish)

Pushups

Pushups are a great alternative to work your chest muscles if you don't have anywhere to do the dumbbell press. Many women have trouble performing push-ups because their upper body isn't strong enough to support their weight. What they don't know is that you can vary the position of your body to match your strength level. The important thing in a push-up is to perform a full range of motion — all the way down until your nose and chest practically touch the floor, and then all the way back up. If you can't go all the way down, your body is telling you to try a less challenging push-up position. Your strength will gradually increase, allowing you to move on to the harder varieties.

Push-Up Level 1: Wall Push-Up

Stand about two feet away from a wall and place your hands on the wall about shoulder height and shoulder width apart. Slowly lean in toward the wall and then push away. Too easy? Then try level 2.

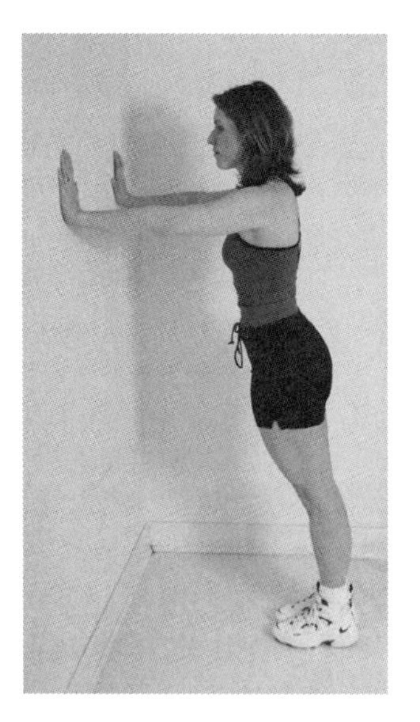

Wall Push-up (start)

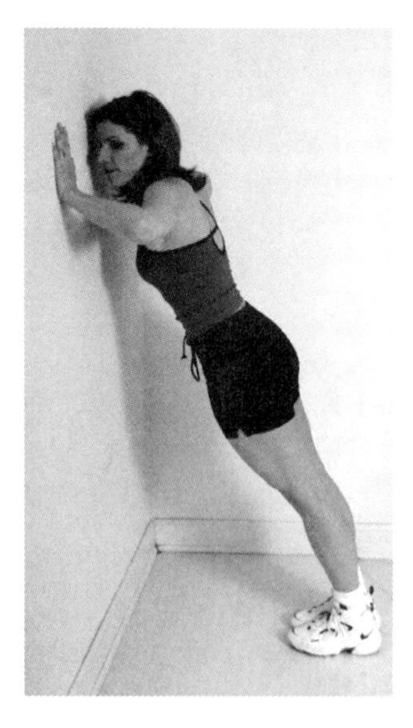

Wall Push-up (finish)

Push-Up Level 2: Floor Push-Up with Hips Bent 90 Degrees

Begin on your hands and knees. Your hips and shoulder joints are bent about 90 degrees, so that your body looks almost like a card table. Lower your head, shoulders, and chest to the floor, leaving your hips in the air so that your full body weight isn't going into the push-up. Push back up to starting position. Too easy? As you lower your head, shoulders, and chest, allow your body to tip forward, releasing more of your body weight into the push-up. Push back to starting position. Still too easy? Try level 3 with a straight body.

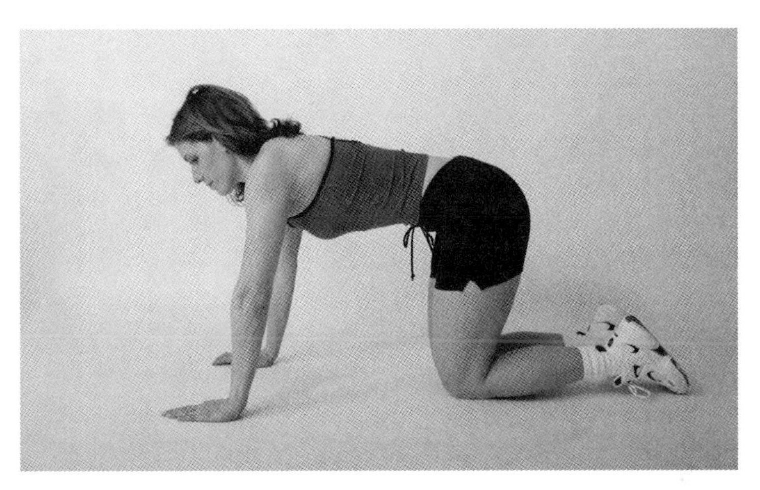

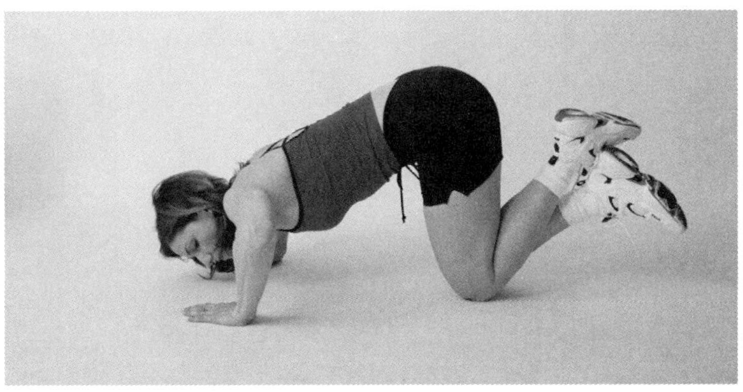

Push-up Level 2 (start and finish)

Push-Up Level 3: Floor Push Up with a Straight Body

This is the push-up that you most commonly see, but that very few women can actually perform correctly unless they already have a good bit of upper body strength. Begin on your hands and knees, except move your hands further away from your knees and straighten your hips so that your body forms a straight diagonal line from your head to your knees. Slowly lower your body toward the floor, keeping your body completely straight as you go. When you get to the bottom, your nose, chest, and stomach should all be close to the floor. Push back to starting position while keeping your body straight as a board. (If you can't go all the way down to the floor or can't keep your body straight on the way back up, you probably need to go back to push-up level 2.)

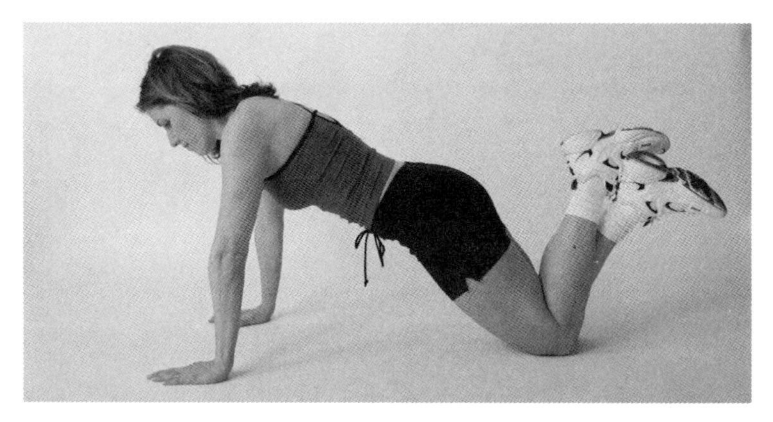

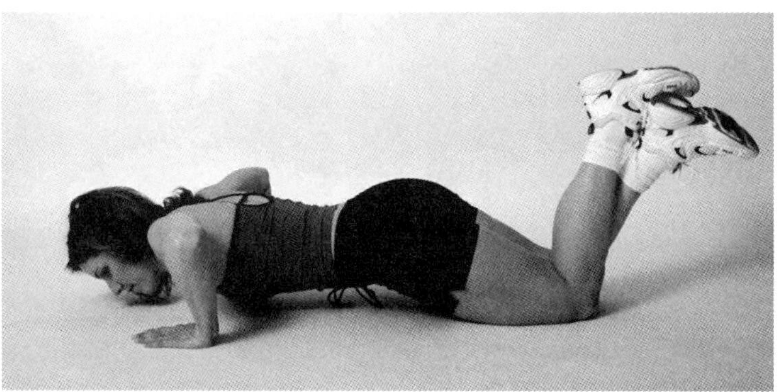

Push-up Level 3 (start and finish)

2. Seated Tubing Row (back)

Sit on the floor with your feet wider than shoulder width apart and your knees slightly bent. Wrap the tubing around the instep portion of both shoes. (Don't try this barefoot — ouch!) Criss-cross the tubing, forming an "X", and then hold the tubing itself, as opposed to the handles. (When you hold the handles, you'll find there is too much slack in the tubing, making the exercise too easy.) Pull your elbows back, being conscious to squeeze your shoulder blades together. Slowly return to the starting position.

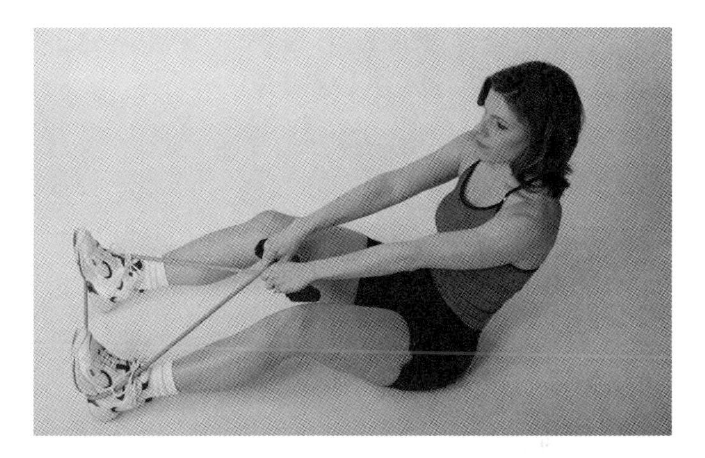

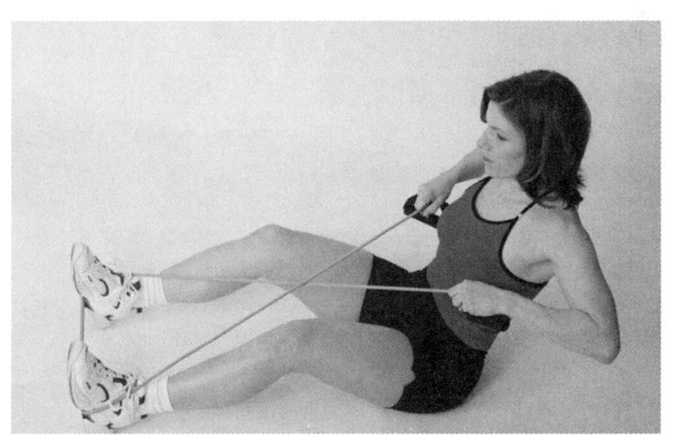

Seated Tubing Row (start and finish)

3. Dumbbell Side Raise (shoulders)

Stand, holding dumbbells in front of your body, palms facing each other. Slowly lift your arms up to the side until they are horizontal, keeping your elbows slightly bent. Your wrists should remain straight. When you get to the top, your wrists and elbows should be the same height, with your palms facing the floor. Slowly lower down to the starting position. If the dumbbells are too heavy, you won't be able to keep elbows and wrists on level, nor your palms facing down. You also want to avoid arching your back, which can happen if the dumbbells are too heavy. Think of the ending position as that of a male gymnast in the rings or imagine yourself holding a bucket in each hand. If your arms twist so that your palms no longer face the floor, you will spill your buckets of water.

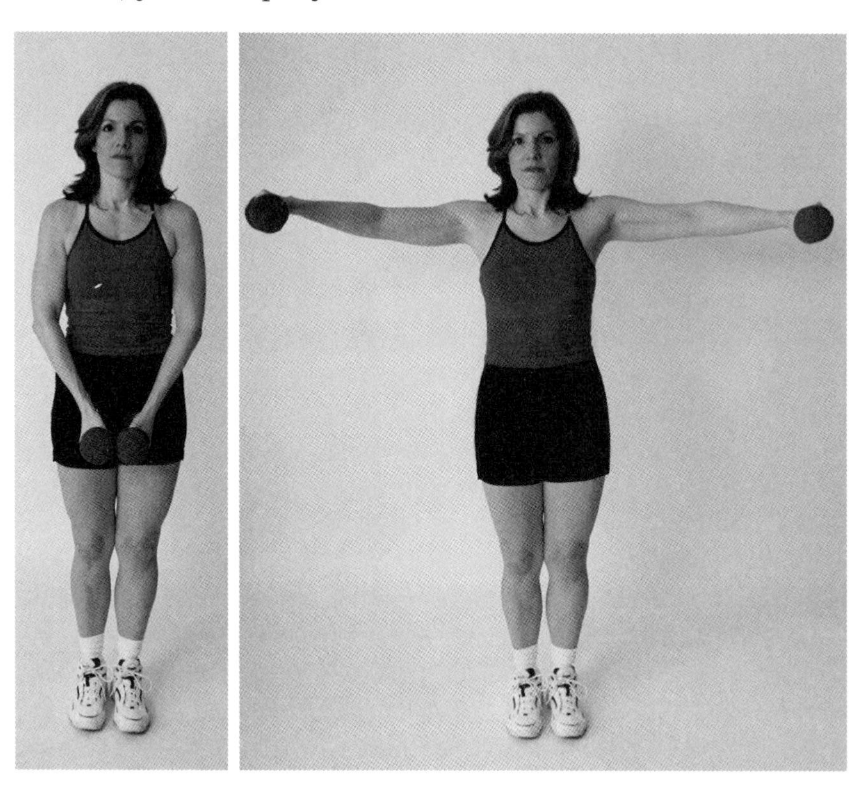

Dumbbell Side Raise (start and finish)

4. Bicep Curl (biceps/front of arm)

Begin with your arms at your sides with your palms facing front. Begin bending one elbow, so that when you end, your palm is facing your chest in front. Return to starting position and then begin the other arm. To make it more challenging (and go quicker!), you can do both arms at the same time. Regardless, be sure that you always go from an entirely straight arm to a completely bent elbow joint and don't use momentum to swing the dumbbell up. When you lower your arm back down, the temptation is to stop and start coming back up before your elbow is completely straight. That's the easy way out! Keep yourself honest by going all the way down and all the way up. If you can't go all the way down before coming back up or you start arching your back, the weight is probably too heavy.

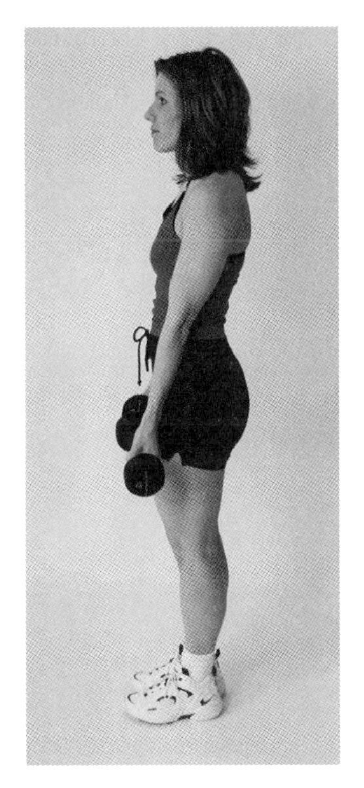

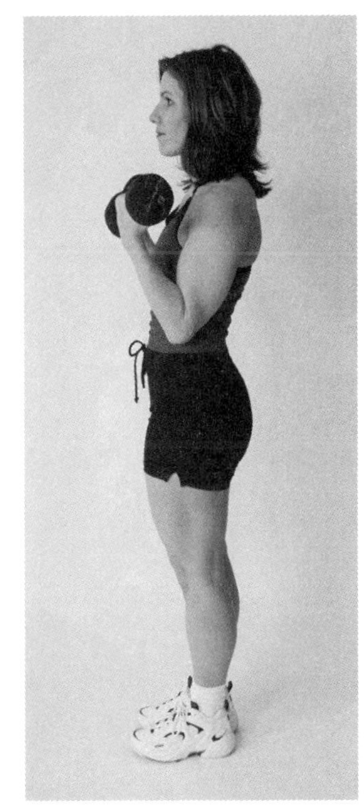

Bicep Curl (start and finish)

5. Overhead Tricep Extension with a Dumbbell (triceps/back of arm)

Hold one dumbbell overhead, as pictured below. Notice that you are not holding the middle of the dumbbell, but rather, you slip the middle part between your thumb and index finger of both hands, and then grip the end of the dumbbell. Keep your elbows close to your head. Slowly bend your elbows so that the dumbbell drops quite low behind your head. Then, straighten your elbows again to return the dumbbell to the starting position. (When returning to the starting position, be sure that you are not moving your shoulder joints, which would throw the entire movement forward. Only move your elbow joints.)

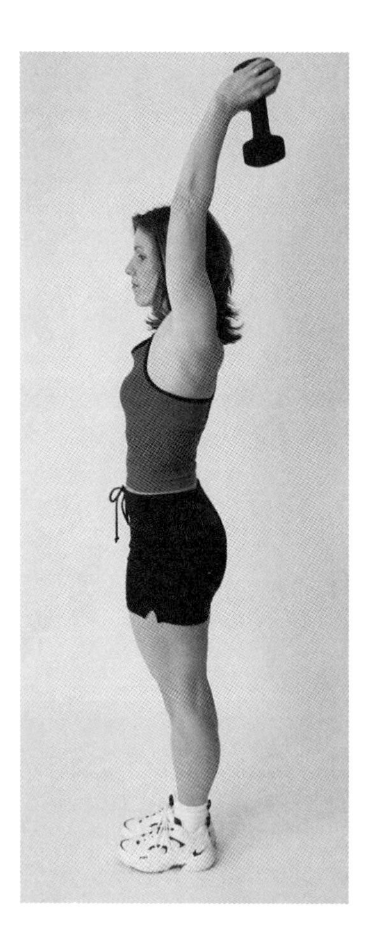

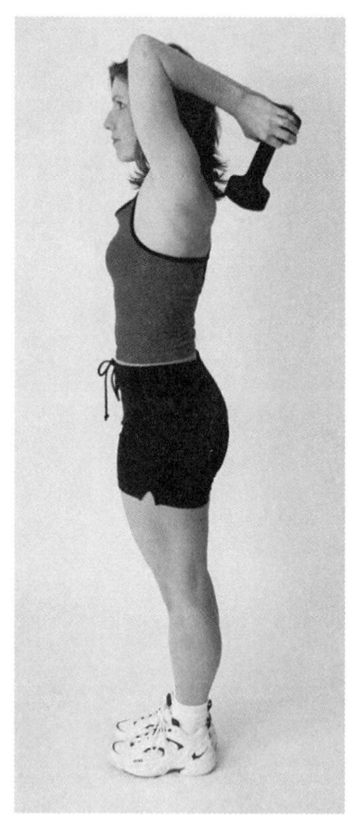

Overhead Tricep Extension (start and finish)

6. Ball Squat or Dumbbell Squat (quadriceps/front of thigh and gluteus maximus/rear end)

The squat is one of my favorite exercises. It's a great way to work both your thighs and rear end at the same time. The ball squat is great for beginners because it is less intense and easier to perform correctly because the ball guides you through the correct range of motion. Dumbbell squats are a little more advanced, requiring more effort to maintain the proper form. Pay careful attention to the instructions below because performing squats incorrectly can put your knees at risk for injury. Try the ball squat first and if it's too easy, move on to the dumbbell squat.

The Ball Squat

Find a wall surface that is flat and bare (no doorknobs, light switches, or picture frames!). Place the ball between you and the wall, about waist height and then put your back to the ball. Press the small of your back firmly against the ball. It should feel like the ball "fits" comfortably in the arch of your back. Adjust your feet so that they are about shoulder-width apart and parallel to each other. Make sure your feet are also several feet away from the wall. If your feet are too close to the wall, your knees will jut out uncomfortably once you begin the motion. If this happens to you, move your feet a few more inches away from the wall and try again. It may take a few tries to find the right foot placement for you based on your height.

The Motion

Slowly begin squatting down by bending your knees and "curling your tailbone under the ball" until your thighs are almost parallel to the ground (approaching a 90 degree bend at the knee joint). Your lower leg should remain fairly vertical, which keeps your knees right over your ankles, not jutting out past your toes. Focus on keeping contact with the ball and avoid leaning forward. Once you get to the "bottom" of the range of motion, push straight back up to your starting position. The ball should roll with you right back to its starting position at the small of your back.

How Far Down?

Knowing how far down to go is important and may take some practice. For some people, going all the way down to "parallel" is uncomfortable. You may only go half that distance and that's okay. You may find that as you build strength, you can gradually go further down. Pay attention to what your knees are telling you and only perform the exercise through the range of motion that is comfortable for you. (Note to over-achievers: "Parallel" is the most advanced stopping point. It is never advisable to go *past* the parallel point, as this is stressful for your knee joints.)

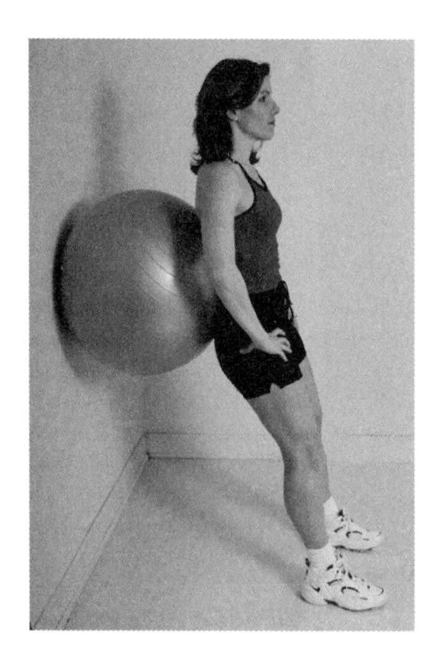

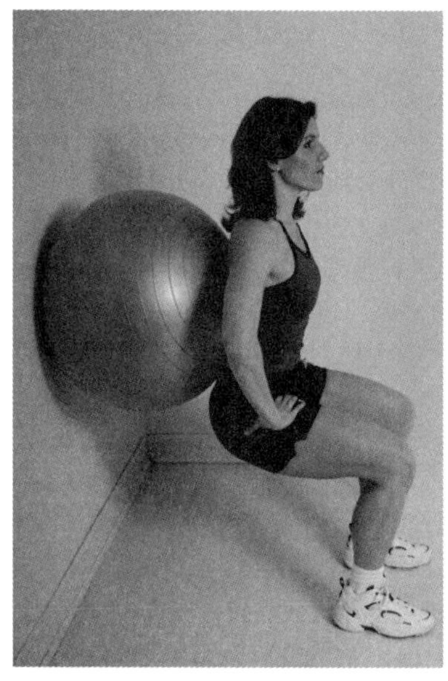

Ball Squat (start and finish)

Note: If the ball slips and starts to fall to the ground, you are performing the exercise incorrectly. Check to see if you are either leaning forward, not pressing the small of your back into the ball, and/or not curling your tailbone under the ball as you go down.

A Few Words of Caution about Squats

Stop if you feel pain, especially in your knees. You may want to double check to make sure you are using the correct form. But even performed correctly, squats may not be for you. Listen to your body and if it hurts, don't do it.

Dumbbell Squats

Stand with feet slightly wider than shoulder-width apart. Brace the dumbbells on your shoulders as pictured below. (Once you are experienced, you will probably use your heaviest dumbbells for this exercise. But when you're just starting out, begin with light dumbbells or no weights at all until you get the hang of it.) Slowly lower down, while focusing on sticking your butt out (I know that sounds weird!), rather than focusing on bending your knees. Try to keep your chest up (you're not taking a bow here), and in doing so, your back will need to arch slightly. The goal is to lower down until your thighs are almost parallel to the floor without letting your knees jut out past your toes. This means that your ankle joints aren't bending at all. Once again, don't go past the parallel point. When you start coming back up, thrust your hips forward in a subtle way so that your body is straight once again.

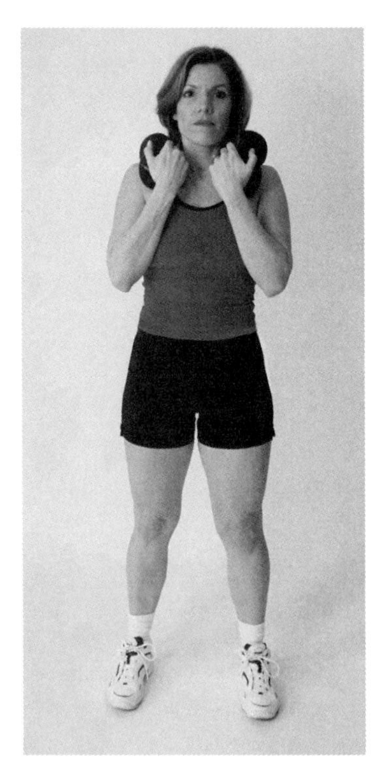

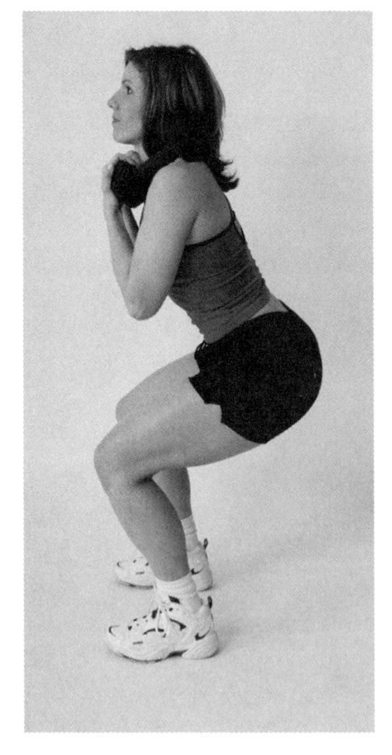

Dumbball Squat (start and finish)

7. Ball Hamstring Curl (hamstrings/back of thigh)

This is a fun exercise that may take a little practice at first in order to keep your balance! Lie on the floor on your back, with your calves and ankles propped up on the ball. If the ball is too close to you (under your knees), you won't have enough room to let the ball roll. If the ball is too far away from you (under your ankles and feet only), it will probably slip away. Brace yourself with your arms pressing down on the floor and lift up your hips. (This is where you may need to practice your balance!) Dig your heels into the ball and roll the ball toward your rear end, then roll back out. You may need to occasionally re-position your feet if the ball starts slipping away from you.

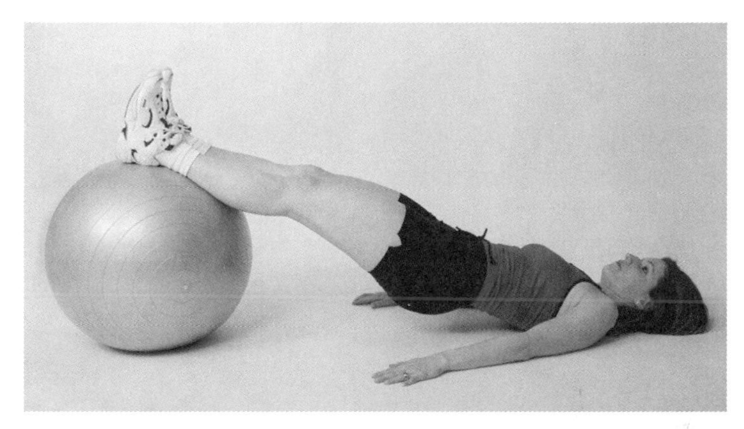

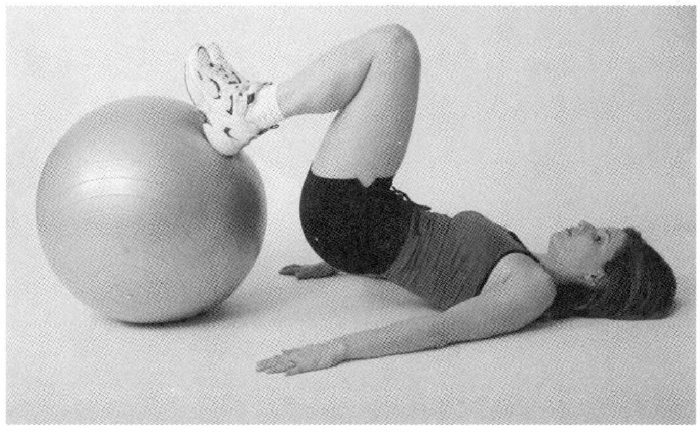

Ball Hamstring Curl (start and finish)

8. Inner Thigh Ball Squeeze (inner thigh)

Approach the ball from behind and carefully sit on it. Roll forward slightly until your hip joint is completely straight. (Your knees are pointing down, not forward and your feet are behind you.) If you fall off the front of the ball, try again but this time start farther back! Once you've got a comfortable position, simply squeeze the ball with your thighs and release. I like to finish with an extended squeeze of 10 or more seconds!

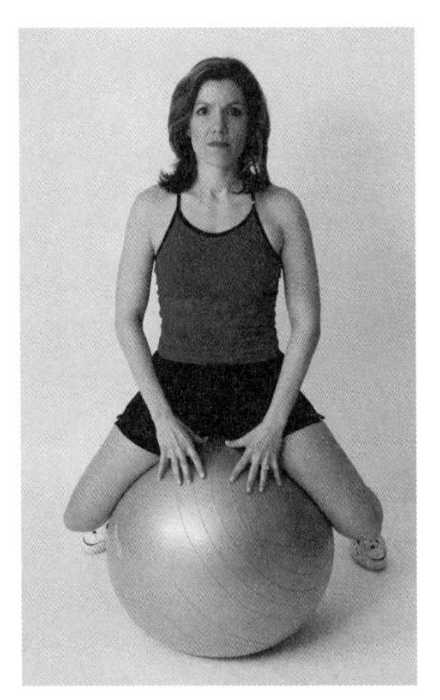

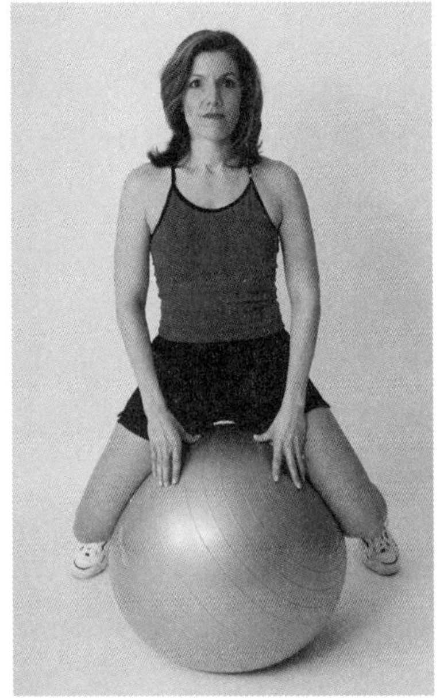

Inner Thigh Ball Squeeze (start and finish)

9. Hip Abduction with Tubing (hips)

Lie on your back on the floor, with the tubing around your feet. Be sure that the tubing is securely caught in the notch of your shoe at the instep. Your legs are overhead, but angled down a bit (not straight up), and your knees are slightly bent. You'll want about 6-10 inches of tubing between your feet. If you feel any cramping in your hip muscles, try angling your legs down even farther. Open and close your legs from the hip joint. Each time you press out, the tubing will stretch and apply a resistance to your hip muscles doing the work. Press out and release back in as many times as you can. I like to finish with holding in the out position for 10 or more seconds!

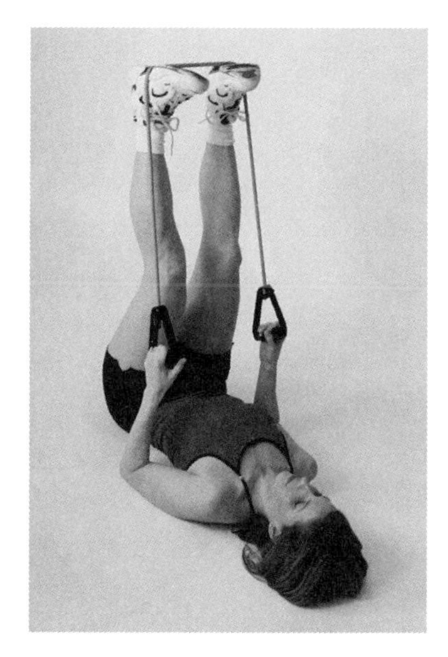

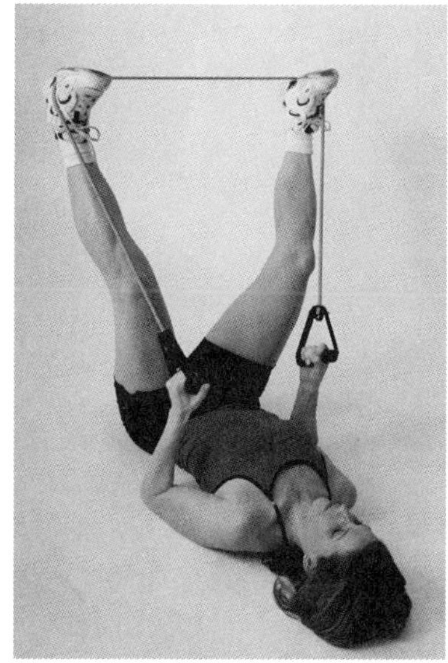

Hip Abduction (start and finish)

10. Crunches (abdominal muscles)

Lie on the floor on your back, with your knees bent and your feet flat on the floor. Your hands can be either crossed over your chest or placed lightly behind your head (not behind your neck). Slowly lift your head and shoulders off the floor until you feel your shoulder blades come off the floor, and then slowly return to the starting position. Be sure to keep your head and neck relaxed during the movement — don't jut your chin up toward the ceiling OR tuck your chin to your chest. Just allow it to remain neutral and natural as you curl up and down. How many crunches should you do? That will depend directly on how strong your abdominal muscles are! You may start with 5, 10, 20 or even 50 crunches. See how you feel and stop when your stomach muscles feel fatigued. Over a period of time, you will be able to do more and more crunches. That will also tell you that you may be ready for more advanced abdominal strengthening exercises!

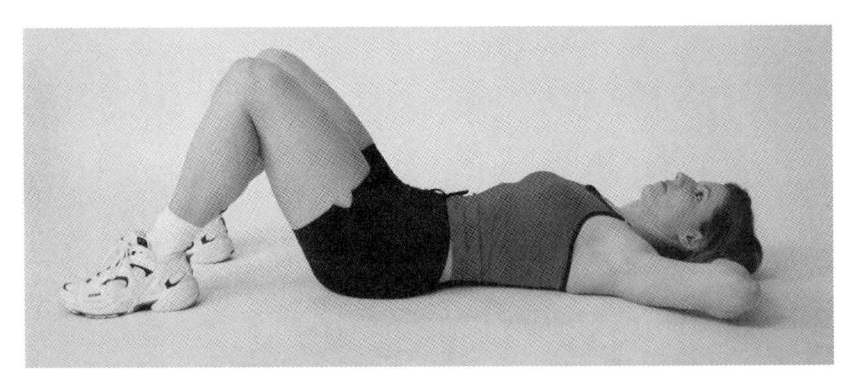

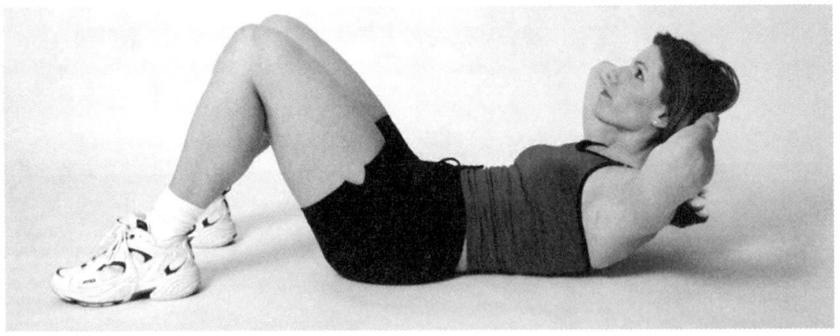

Crunches (start and finish)

The Busy Mom's Intermediate and Advanced Plan Stretches

For the Intermediate Exercise Plan, you need only perform the following first four stretches listed:

- ✔ Calf Stretch
- ✔ Quadriceps stretch
- ✔ Lower back stretch
- ✔ Hamstring stretch

These four stretches target muscles that can most benefit from stretching. To keep things simplified, you can wait until the very end of your cardio or weight training routine to do these stretches. Or, if you prefer, you can perform each stretch after working the corresponding muscle. If that's the case, you may end up adding in the rest of the stretches listed for the Advanced Exercise Plan. The choice is yours.

For the Advanced Exercise Plan, you will want to perform each of the listed stretches after working that particular muscle group.

Calf Stretch

Stand with your feet together and then take a large step back with one foot. Bend the front knee just a bit until you feel the stretch in the calf of your back leg. Make sure your front knee doesn't jut out past your toe and that the heel of your back foot stays on the floor.

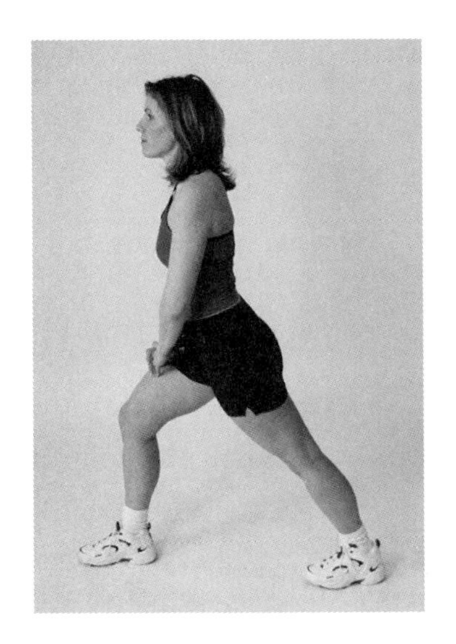

Calf Stretch

Quadriceps Stretch

Stand on one foot and hold the other foot up behind you as pictured. Be sure to keep your knees close together.

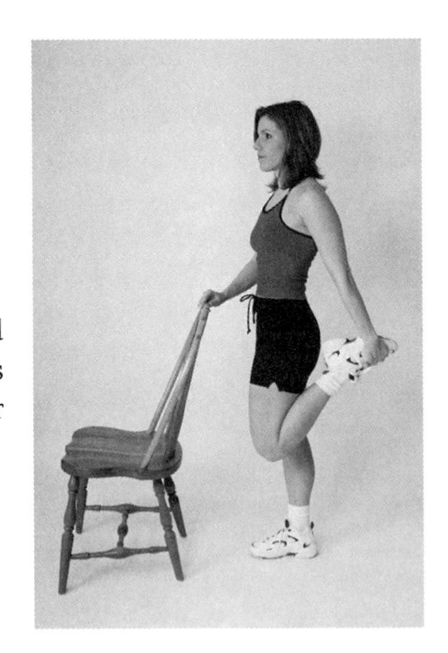

Quadricep Stretch

Lower Back Stretch

Lie on your back on the floor and pull both knees to your chest. Hold both knees to your chest with your hands, clasping your hands under your knees if possible.

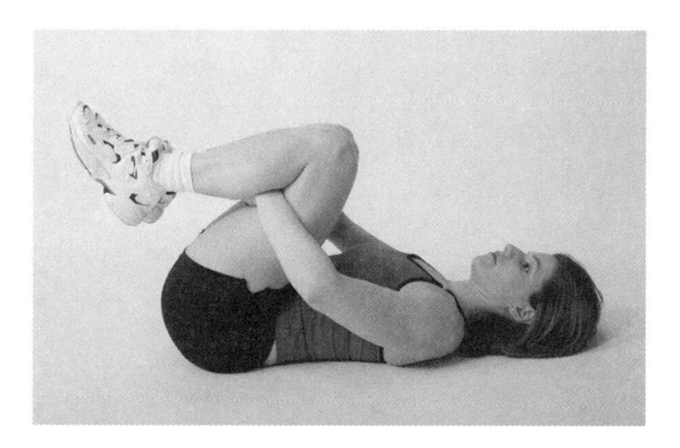

Lower Back Stretch

Hamstring Stretch

While lying on the floor on your back, keep one leg bent with your foot flat on the floor. Extend the other leg up and pull towards your body with your hands, keeping your knee slightly bent and your lower back pressed to the floor. Switch.

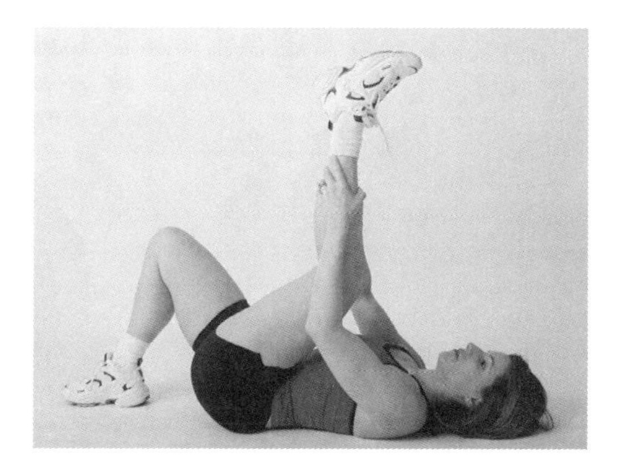

Hamstring Stretch

Inner Thigh Stretch

Stand with your legs wide apart and toes facing straight ahead. Shift your weight to one side and hold. Then switch.

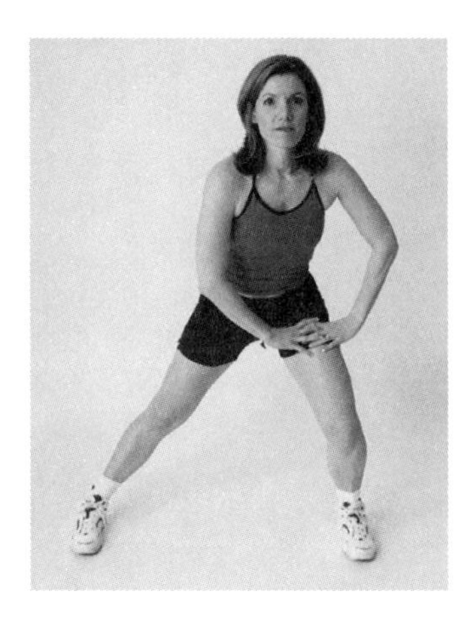

Inner Thigh Stretch

Hip Stretch

Lie on your back with your knees bent and feet flat on the floor. Place your right foot on your left knee, then lift your left leg off the floor and clasp your hands together under your left knee. Switch.

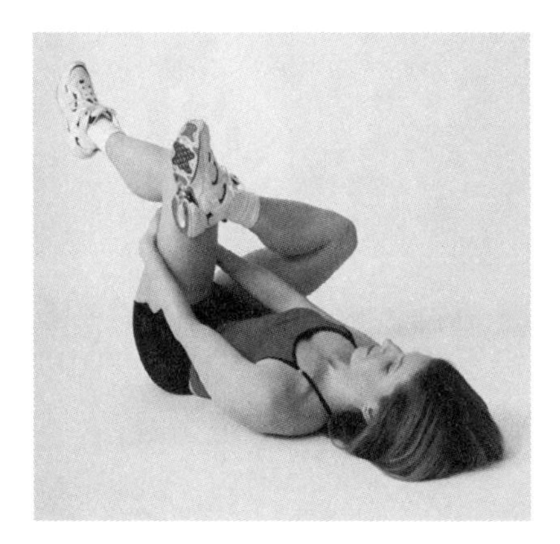

Hip Stretch

Chest Stretch

Let your arms fall open wide. Pull your arms back, squeezing shoulder blades together.

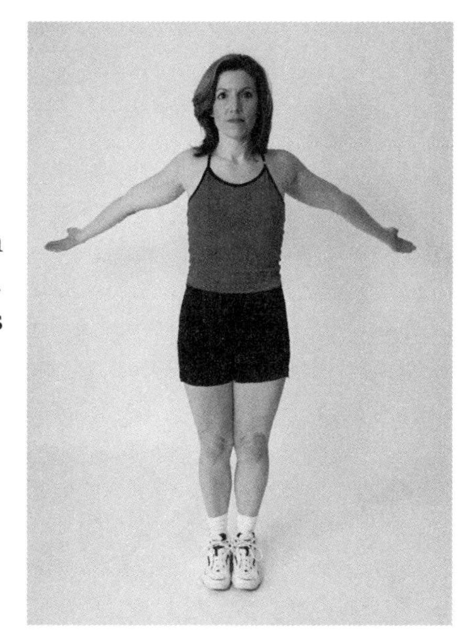

Chest Stretch

Upper Back Stretch

While standing, clasp your hands out in front of you with straight arms and press out, rounding your upper back.

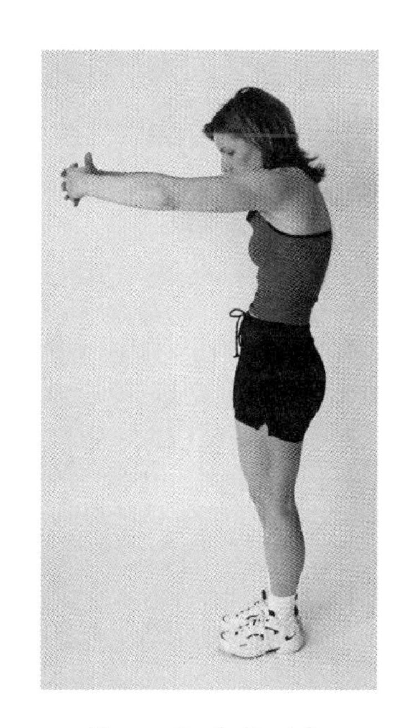

Upper Back Stretch

Shoulder Stretch

Grab your left arm with your right hand and pull it across your chest, pressing it toward your body. Switch.

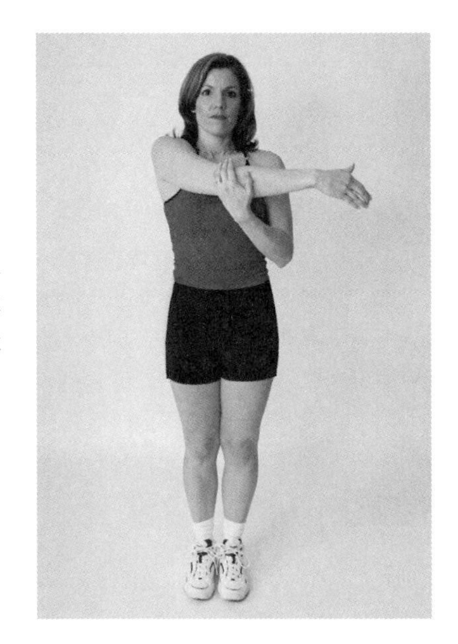

Shoulder Stretch

Bicep Stretch

Hang your arms down at your sides and press down and out with the heel of your hands.

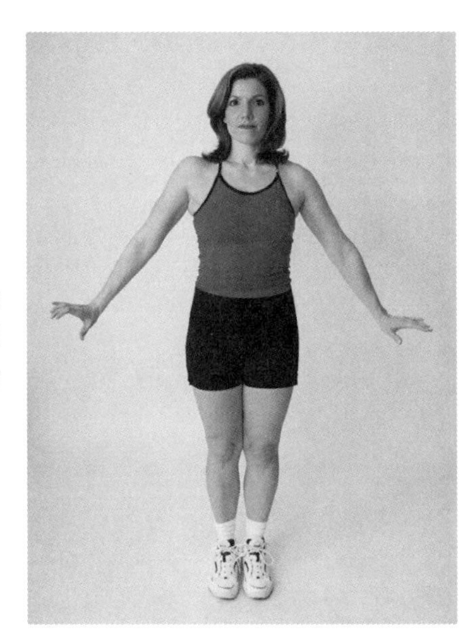

Bicep Stretch

Tricep Stretch

Lift one arm overhead, elbow bent, with your hand hanging down your back. With the fingertips of your opposite hand, pull back just above the elbow. Switch.

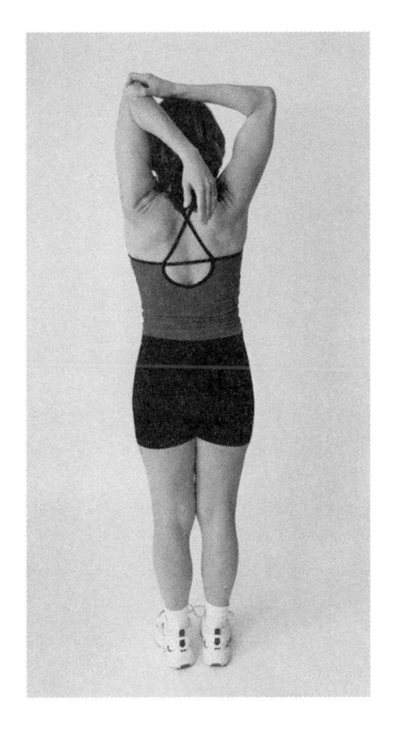

Tricep Stretch

Appendix 3

Prenatal and Postnatal Fitness

Whether this is your first baby or the latest addition to your brood, pregnancy is a special time. You're happy! You have so may hopes and dreams for this new chapter in your life. There is another person inside of you! Suddenly, everything you do with your body also affects another person. It takes some getting used to! You drive differently; you go up and down stairs just a little more carefully . . . you know there are probably some special guidelines for exercising during pregnancy. Thankfully, we've come a long way from the times when people assumed pregnancy was a "delicate" condition and that most any exertion could be harmful to the baby. Those who did exercise may have been met with raised eyebrows for being so selfish while being asked "Are you sure that's okay to do?" Exercising moms-to-be have been vindicated in recent years — current research shows that not only is exercise not harmful to the baby, for almost all healthy pregnant women with normal, low-risk pregnancies it's better for the baby than not exercising. If your doctor has told you that your pregnancy is high risk, then you will need to follow specific guidelines given to you by your health-care professional. In any case, however, it is always a good idea to discuss your plans to exercise with your doctor prior to starting an exercise routine while pregnant (or at any other time, in life, for that matter).

Take a look at the following benefits you have to gain by exercising during pregnancy:

- ✔ Helps prevent excessive weight gain
- ✔ Helps manage stress
- ✔ Maintains cardiovascular and muscular fitness
- ✔ Improves balance and coordination (some moms feel clumsy as their bellies grow!)
- ✔ Lessens back pain
- ✔ Improves circulation
- ✔ Helps prevent gestational diabetes
- ✔ Helps to maintain the strength and integrity of the abdominal muscles
- ✔ Improves the support of pelvic organs
- ✔ Decreases the minor discomforts of pregnancy (varicose veins, leg cramps, swelling, constipation)
- ✔ Increases energy
- ✔ Improves your strength and endurance for labor
- ✔ Returns you to your pre-pregnancy weight sooner

So now that you know you *should* probably be exercising through your pregnancy, the questions become . . .

What kinds of exercises are best for me?

What kinds of exercises should be avoided?

How much should I do and how do I know when it's too much?

How do I make sure I am doing the exercises safely and correctly during this important time?

Normal Physiological Changes During Pregnancy

Before we discuss how exercise impacts your baby and your pregnant body, let's first look at the normal physiological changes that happen in your body during pregnancy. It's important to understand all of these changes so that you can see that your body is already working very hard to grow and nurture your baby, even when you are just sitting or lying down!

- Your blood volume increases by almost double, with much of the increased circulation going to your baby for growth.
- Hormonal changes may cause your ligaments to be somewhat looser, which may cause your joints to become less stable.
- Your center of gravity changes as your belly grows.
- With your growing belly weighing down in front, your lower back muscles come under greater strain.
- Because the baby is at your core and has no access to the surface for heat dissipation, your baby's body temperature is higher than your body temperature.
- Your abdominal muscles stretch as your belly grows.
- Your pelvic organs press down on your pelvic floor muscles with increasing pressure.
- During the third trimester of pregnancy, your body is capable of creating more fat cells. This is often the reason that losing "baby weight" can be more difficult than losing weight at other times in your life. Keeping weight gain to a minimum (typically 25-35 pounds total), especially during this third trimester is important to prevent new fat cells from forming. (The first year of life and the adolescent growth spurt are generally the only other times when your body actually makes more fat cells. At all other times in life, unless there is an extremely large and sudden weight gain, additional weight is usually due to increased size of existing fat cells.)

- When lying on your back, the weight of the developing baby can compress the vena cava (the large vein returning blood to the heart), causing decreased oxygen flow to you and the baby. Many times, this is accompanied by lightheadedness, but not all the time.

Exercise Recommendations During Pregnancy

✔ According to the American College of Obstetrics and Gynecology (ACOG), in the absence of medical or obstetric complications, 30 minutes or more of moderate exercise per day on most, if not all, days of the week is recommended for pregnant women.

✔ Low impact aerobic exercise can be continued throughout pregnancy, with many women continuing until the day before they deliver. You may have heard to limit your heart rate to 140 beats per minute or less. *This is an outdated recommendation that is no longer endorsed by ACOG.* Perceived exertion is a better indicator of intensity for aerobic exercise during pregnancy. Aim for a "somewhat hard" feeling and trust your instincts that you are not overdoing it.

✔ Spend plenty of time (at least 5 minutes) gradually warming up before and cooling down after aerobic exercise.

✔ Weight training can be continued, but it's a good idea to gradually decrease the weights used so that they are lighter than those used pre-pregnancy, for two reasons: 1) your joints may be less stable and 2) to ensure a continuous oxygen supply. You should be able to breathe comfortably throughout the entire exercise. It is important to select a weight that you can lift comfortably the entire range of motion for the entire set. At no point should you be straining to finish a repetition or feel the need to hold your breath.

✔ Do not perform weight exercises or crunches flat on your back. Instead of bench press or dumbbell flies on a flat bench, for example, do them on an incline.

Crunches can also be performed on an incline bench instead of the floor. As your pregnancy progresses, you will find that certain exercises are no longer comfortable. Listen to your body and discontinue those exercises.

- ✔ Include stretching exercises, especially for the lower back muscles. Rather than lying on your back and trying to hold your knees to your chest, try the cat back stretch (round your back up while on your hands and knees) or the "seated back relaxer" described in Chapter 8.

- ✔ **Include Kegel exercises to strengthen the muscles of the pelvic floor.**

  Sagging pelvic organs and urinary incontinence are not dinner party conversation, but they are, unfortunately, a common part of pregnancy. Do you know where your Kegel muscles are? You find them by imagining that you need to urinate and have to "hold" it. You use these muscles to stop and start the flow of urine. *(Note: Don't practice this exercise while you are urinating! This habit puts you at risk for a urinary tract infection by possibly causing urine to flow backward.)* These pelvic floor muscles are under an incredible amount of pressure as your belly grows and presses down on your pelvic floor. Once you've found your Kegel muscles, squeeze (contract) these muscles and hold for 10 seconds if possible. Relax the muscles and repeat up to 10 times every day if possible. Be sure that you are not squeezing your abdominal, inner thigh, or gluteal muscles . . . just the pelvic floor muscles!

- ✔ Drink plenty of water before, during, and after exercise.

- ✔ Listen to your body. Stop exercising if you feel dizzy, uncomfortable, or overly tired.

Exercise Cautions and Restrictions During Pregnancy

While your doctor is the final authority for what you should and should not do while you are pregnant, the following are general recommendations:

- Avoid activities with a high risk of falling or abdominal trauma (such as skiing or horseback riding) or decompression sickness (scuba diving).
- You may find that activities involving jumping, running, bouncing, and other high impact movements are less comfortable as your pregnancy progresses. There is no inherent risk to the baby, but because your joints and connective tissue may be less stable, you will probably be more comfortable with lower impact activities.
- It is a good idea to limit (or proceed with caution) activities that involve a lot of lateral movement (like aerobic dance or step aerobics) because joints may be less stable.
- Avoid exercising outdoors in the high heat and humidity.

  Body temperature increases with exercise, and perspiration allows your body to cool. Your baby, at the core of a woman's body, has a higher body temperature, and has no outside surface from which to sweat and dissipate heat. It is therefore important that you do not become overheated. If you become overheated, your baby's body is even more so, and he or she has no mechanism with which to cool down.
- Avoid lying flat on your back as much as possible after the first trimester. If you have no symptoms of lightheadedness, you may continue until the last trimester or so, if you wish. However, since some studies show that oxygen could be restricted even if you don't feel any symptoms, the most conservative thing would be to lie on an incline when possible.

- Avoid holding your breath and straining (known as the valsalva maneuver), especially when lifting weights. This can cause an increase in blood pressure and decreased oxygen flow.

Warning Signs to Discontinue Exercise While Pregnant

According to ACOG, you should take heed of the below circumstances, which signal you to stop exercising and consult your doctor:

- Vaginal bleeding
- Shortness of breath prior to exertion
- Dizziness
- Headache
- Chest pain
- Muscle weakness
- Calf pain or swelling
- Pre-term labor
- Decreased fetal movement
- Amniotic fluid leakage

Exercising while you are pregnant can be one of the best sanity-savers! Resist the urge to think of this time as a period of indulgence and trepidation. Embrace your growing body and continue to move, move, move! It will feel good and your baby will thank you for all that extra oxygen you are pumping through your body!

Getting Your Body Back into Shape after Baby

When everyone asks how you are doing, of course your answer is "The baby is healthy and that's all we care about!" But, inside you may be wondering, "Will I ever get my old body back? Will my stomach ever be the same again? How can I think about getting back in shape when I can't even get any sleep?" The demands of a newborn leave you bleary-eyed, and the physical changes after having a baby can be tough to manage for even those in the best shape.

While more strenuous exercise will have to wait until the baby is about six weeks old, most women don't have to wait that long (and shouldn't!) before they begin the gentle progression back to their pre-pregnancy exercise routine. In fact, there are several types of exercise that are beneficial starting the first day home from the hospital. Let's talk through the stages as well as keys to full abdominal muscle rehabilitation.

Did you read that right? Yes! I said abdominal muscle *rehabilitation*. Please do *not* think the answer to getting your abs back is to do tons of crunches, starting as early as possible. This can be bad news to your newly traumatized abdominal muscles. The proper exercises and progression of exercise can help you regain as flat of a stomach as possible. By the way, even if your "baby" is 2 years old (or even older), it's not too late to rehabilitate your abdominal muscles.

What about that pesky problem of losing a drop of urine here and there (with a laugh, a sneeze, or a jumping jack)? Has anyone told you that bladder incontinence is just a fact of life after having kids? It does *not* have to be that way! Your pelvic floor muscles have a job to do holding up your internal organs, and they, too, have been traumatized through pregnancy and delivery. Sheila Watkins, of Healthy Moms ® has a great visualization for what your pelvic floor muscles have been through after pregnancy. They are *supposed* to function like a trampoline as they hold your pelvic organs up, but sometimes they more closely resemble a hammock after having kids! What do your pelvic floor muscles look like: a trampoline or a hammock? Kegel exercises are the key to regaining full pelvic floor muscle stability and you can do these exercises anytime and anywhere! Refer back to the section "Exercise Recommendations During Pregnancy" for instructions on how to do Kegels.

General Physical Changes Postpartum

Let's first review some of the changes that your body goes through postpartum before you add exercise to the mix:

1. Your abdominal and pelvic organs gradually rearrange to pre-pregnancy locations.
2. Your spine gradually returns to pre-pregnancy alignment (during pregnancy, the S curve of the spine had deepened and the center of gravity had shifted).
3. Your uterus shrinks from 2.5 pounds back to about 2.5 ounces.
4. Your vaginal bleeding fades from red to brown to yellow before it stops completely.
5. Your relaxed ligaments from the hormone changes during pregnancy will continue for 6-16 weeks before going back to normal.
6. You may experience sore or engorged breasts (a supportive sports bra or nursing before exercise will minimize discomfort).
7. Your abdominal muscles will be lengthened and weakened.
8. Your pelvic floor muscles are weakened and the tissue is bruised and swollen.

More About Abdominal Muscle Changes

After pregnancy, your abdominal muscles are both stretched and weakened. The muscle fibers have been lengthened; therefore they must be *shortened before they are strengthened* (see the exercises on the following page). Otherwise, the outcome could be stronger muscles that "bunch up" and thus continue to stick out. In addition, many women experience diastasis recti (a separation of the abdominal muscles down the middle). A diastasis recti can be troublesome. Usually a minor separation can be improved with some of the exercises outlined here. Larger separations may need surgical attention, especially if you experience lower back pain or a hernia. Be sure to consult with your physician if you think you have a substantial separation.

Exercises that Can Be Done from Days 1–14 Postpartum

While you won't be doing very much in the way of exercise for the first 2 weeks, there are some things that are definitely valuable and don't take a lot of time. You'll want to engage the abdominal muscles and pelvic floor muscles as soon as possible. The entire area has been traumatized, including the nerve pathways to those muscles. One of the best ways to reinforce those nerve pathways and remind those muscles how to contract is to do isometric exercises — the kind where you contract and *hold* a position for 10–30 seconds. Here are two simple exercises that I recommend from day one:

1. *Shorten the abdominal muscles by "sucking in" or "pulling your naval to your spine."*

   While lying on your back, suck in your abdominal muscles while visualizing that you are pulling your naval to your spine. Start by holding the position for just a few seconds and progress to holding it up to 30 seconds. You can do this every day.

2. *Strengthen the pelvic floor muscles by doing Kegel exercises*

   When you first begin doing Kegels after delivery, you may not even feel what you are doing! Those muscles and nerve pathways are traumatized so the stimulus will be valuable, even if you can't immediately tell what you are doing. Keep at it, starting with just a few contractions, holding each contraction for just a few seconds. Build up to 10 repetitions, holding each one for 10 seconds.

Gradual Return to Regular Exercise Starting At Two Weeks Postpartum

Many moms are anxious to return to exercise. Others love the "free pass" of waiting until the traditional recommendation of six weeks postpartum. Caregiver advice now varies. For a vaginal delivery, you should wait a minimum of 10–14 days postpartum for any exercise beyond the two exercises described previously. (Wait until bleeding is brownish and mostly done; if it returns to bright red, you've probably done too much too soon.) If you begin exercising as soon as 10-14 days, be sure to gradually build back up. You'll want to start with a modified program and save the higher intensity/high impact activities for the 6-week mark. If you can find a specialty postnatal fitness class near you, you'll benefit from special instruction as well as camaraderie and support.

Exercise Progression Tips for Postnatal Moms

1. Abdominal Shortening Exercises

Hopefully you have been doing these since day one. If not, start them as soon as possible and keep at it. First "suck it in" and then pretend you are trying to "zip up" a pair of too-tight jeans. (Build up to holding for 10 seconds each repetition. Do as many repetitions as you can or would like to do.)

2. Check for Diastasis Recti

Some time after the third day, check to see how much the abdominal muscles have separated down the middle (diastasis recti). Lie down on your back with your knees bent. Press your fingers firmly into the area around your naval while slowly raising your head and shoulders off the floor. How many fingers fit into the "gap"? A slight gap (~1 finger fits in the gap) is usually described as tissue slackness that will close on its own. A wider gap (~2 fingers width) will require special attention with the corrective exercise described next.

3. Corrective Exercises for Closing the Abdominal Gap

All postpartum moms should do these exercises, but how wide the diastasis recti is will determine how quickly you pass this stage. Remember that progressing to regular crunches before doing corrective exercises or before your abdominal muscles are strong enough could make the gap worse. Keep checking the gap and gradually move through the stages as long as the gap doesn't worsen.

a. *"Tuck It In" while bracing the abdominal muscles*

Lie on your back with your knees bent. Cross your hands at your waist and guide the abdominal muscles toward the midline of your body to stabilize them. Inhale. Then slowly exhale and "pull naval to spine" while using your hands to brace the two sides of the diastasis recti together. Return to starting position. Hold for up to 10 seconds and repeat up to 10 times.

b. *Progress to "Tuck It In" while adding a head lift.*

This stage involves lifting the head only; do not yet raise shoulders as this can make the gap worse if your muscles are not yet ready for it. You will do this exercise while continuing the practice of bracing the abdominal muscles with your hands. Try to do 50 repetitions per day. Consistency is important here to help the muscles gradually strengthen with support.

c. *Progress to "Tuck It In" while adding shoulder lifts*

You should not do this exercise until your diastasis (see item 2 on previous page) is less than one finger width. Recovery time will vary from person to person. At first, you will again employ the abdominal muscle bracing technique with your hands. Return to head lifts if the gap increases. Try to build up to 50 repetitions per day.

4. Kegels

Keep doing lots of Kegels. Those pelvic floor muscles need the stimulation to heal, prevent sagging, and prevent leakage of urine. Surely it's worth it! Work up to 10 times, 10 seconds each.

5. Cardiovascular Exercise

Walking is the best cardiovascular exercise to begin with. Mild walking is a good idea from day one; *exercise* walking at a brisk pace should probably wait until after 10–14 days postpartum or when the bleeding subsides as discussed earlier. Gradually increase your intensity and duration. Using a stair machine, participating in step aerobics, or cycling can gradually be added at about 4 weeks. High impact activities, such as running, can be added after 6 weeks.

6. Weight Training

After the 10–14 days postpartum, gradually rebuild to your previous routine. Start with just a few exercises, using lighter weights than normal and paying special attention to your form and body alignment. Keep in mind that your ligaments may still be slightly relaxed so progress with caution. In addition, because your abdominal muscles are weakened, you may find that you experience back pain or other discomforts during some weight-training exercises for a while until you regain some of your abdominal strength and core stability. Proceed carefully and listen to your body.

7. Cesarean Birth Recovery

Gentle abdominal contractions, such as "pulling your naval to your spine" can be helpful to promote healing and muscle recovery. All of the other recommendations still apply, with the exception of a longer time frame before recovery and before progressing through the stages. You will want to wait 3–4 weeks (instead of 2) before doing the modified exercises described in this chapter and up to 8 weeks (instead of 6) before resuming regular/pre-pregnancy levels of exercise.

Remember that your goals in the beginning stages of postpartum exercise are to heal your body, improve your health and gradually ramp back up to your pre-pregnancy exercise habits. With a new little baby in the house, you will have lots of other demands and less sleep. Exercise will help give you the energy you need, but don't put undue pressure on yourself to do more than you are ready for. There will be plenty of time as the baby grows and you settle into your new daily routine. For more information about prenatal and postnatal fitness, you'll want to check out www.healthymomsfitness.com. Good luck!

Appendix 4

Words of Wisdom from Busy Moms Who Are Making It Work ... and Other Motivational Thoughts

What do they have that I don't have?

You may still be struggling to find your fitness solution. You may still be waiting for the click that turns on your internal motivation to exercise regularly. Why not pick up a few pointers or a little food for thought from those who are successful in what you are striving for? There may be something in the following collection that really speaks to you.

At first I felt really guilty taking time away from the kids. I called working out my "selfish hour." It was an hour away from the phones, paperwork, and my children wanting undivided attention. However, the more I thought about it, the more I realized that it wasn't selfish. Working out gives me more energy and makes me happy, which makes me a better mom. I have more energy and do more with my kids.
~ Tracy, mother of three

Exercise improves my mood, gives me energy and helps me maintain my weight. I try to set goals for myself for fitness and strength and then exceed them. The hardest part I find is trying to fit a workout into a day that's already packed with meetings, activities and now, my children's different schedules. But I believe that exercise has become more important to me since I've had children. In seeing their parents exercise, my children have come to view exercise as important for their health as well. ~ Andrea, mother of two

My motivation to keep exercise a part of my daily life has changed over the years. I still exercise to "look good," but have discovered that I just feel so much better when I take the time to take care of myself. As a mother of two young boys, I need lots of energy and time to recharge. Exercise is my answer. ~ Chris, mother of two

I exercise because I just don't feel well if I don't. I need to run, jump, move, sweat and stretch to really feel alive! It energizes me and gives me a more positive and cheerful attitude toward life in general. ~ Jeanne, mother of one

Step class is the one hour out of my day that I don't have to talk to anybody. I don't have to tell anybody what to do — someone tells me! I can listen to good music (not Barney), and the more I sweat, the more I feel the stress pouring out of my body! ~ Abby, mother of three

Many things motivate me to exercise so it's tough to boil it down. I would say the number one reason is because I feel much better physically and emotionally after I exercise. I have more energy and a more positive outlook after I exercise. I prefer to exercise in the morning because I am most efficient and energetic after I exercise. Exercise has become part of my everyday (or almost every day) life. I don't even think about it, I just do it. Being a working mother with a very hectic lifestyle, I look at exercise time as "my time." It is the one hour of the day that I can do something for me that I know is good for me and I enjoy. I only have limited time each day to do something I want to do for myself. I make exercise my priority for that one hour because it is important to me. The rest of the day and night is dedicated to family, work, etc. I couldn't imagine living life without exercise! ~ Susie, mother of two

I have always found using exercise equipment terminally boring. Someone aptly called it "gerbilling". I have never been able to read while walking on the treadmill, I tried watching TV but the shows wear thin after awhile and I hated the commercials. I listened to tapes of music and that helped for a while. Now I have a system I love. I have a good set of headphones that I plug into the TV set so I don't even hear the noise of the treadmill and I watch movies. It works out great. ~ Carol, mother of two

I began running in May 1986. I had left a job that had left me demoralized, and I needed something to get my self-esteem back. I have had struggles with my weight at times in my life, but at that particular time was quite slender, so weight really wasn't part of exercising initially. What I found was a sense of accomplishment. When I first started, to run the five minutes around my court was torture. By October that same year, I ran my first 10 K. It was demonstrable rapid improvement. I've never been a fast runner, but I have pretty good endurance. I have found that I feel much better physically and mentally when I exercise. (I use an exercise bike when it's too cold out, or if I have an injury that keeps me from running). I also have high cholesterol, and regular exercise helps to boost my good cholesterol

(HDL). I like to eat, and running helps to burn those calories. My weight will fluctuate, but stays within an acceptable range for me. I see that as a definite benefit of regular exercise. My job is sedentary; exercise helps to clear my brain and get my blood moving in a way that would never happen in a sedentary job. In addition, as a therapist, I feel an obligation to be a role model for my clients. I recommend exercise to my clients who are dealing with depression and anxiety; research supports the mental health benefits of exercise. I have completed both the Marine Corps Marathon and the JFK 50 miler. Preparation for, and completion of, both events was a totally awesome process. As I said, I've never been fast, but to set a goal such as a long race, and finish it, is tremendously rewarding, and can really be a metaphor for other challenges in life. ~ Mary, mother of two

I have exercised for many years and what motivates me to exercise is that I feel energized and refreshed both physically and mentally. It is almost like an addiction for me because my mind and body both crave exercise! It sounds weird, but it is so true. It makes me feel better mentally as it gets rid of my stress, helps keep my outlook positive, makes me a more patient parent and helps me sleep like a baby at night. Physically, it helps me stay in shape, but honestly, I value most the mental health benefits I gain from it in my busy life of raising a family. I did work professionally for many years prior to having a family and even then, exercise was an important part of my daily living. ~ Lorraine, mother of two

A lot of things motivate me to exercise. For one, I love it. I mean I really love the way it makes me feel when I am done. When I was younger I used to exercise for different reasons, but now I really exercise because it helps with stress. I really exercise for the health of it. It slows down the aging process and I want to be healthy as I get older and show my kids a healthy way of life hoping they will pick up on it. My oldest son exercises everyday so at least he picked up on it; I'm hoping the other three will, as well. I just want to be healthy as I get older and be able to keep up with my kids and grandkids. I don't ever want to be dependent on anyone else. I want to stay strong and fit. ~ Cheryl, mother of four

We all know it. Exercise makes us look and feel better. Yet many of us just don't fit it into our schedules. What's my key to making fitness a priority? It's the reality that a mere 30 minutes of cardiovascular training, Pilates or strength training, five or six days/week makes me feel so energetic I can easily accomplish tasks that overwhelm me when I'm in the "couch potato" mode. It's knowing that 30 minutes of daily movement allows me to release the stress of life. It's the inspiration to eat and live well that comes from squeezing just 180 minutes or 3 hours per week of exercise in my busy schedule. Three hours per week? That's nothing for the benefits of feeling and looking great. I've been consistent for 30 years and see no end in sight. Turns out that all the compliments I get at age 50 are a pretty good incentive too. ~ Leslie, mother of two

Music is a great motivator for me. When I'm in a slump or faced with a problem, I stick on the headphones and get moving. On the treadmill I lose myself in the music and work through the frustration. Now that my children are a little older (5,8,10), my husband and I carve out a little time on the weekends to be outside walking. This gives us a chance to talk, share, and laugh together. The older ones can chose to stay home or join us and my youngest is usually on his bike. We leave our cell phone number with the older ones and stay close to home. It's great for our bodies and our marriage! When I notice that my clothes fit better, my whole mood improves. Exercise helps me be the mother I wish to be. Exercising regularly helps me manage stress, eat healthier, sleep better, and gives me a more positive outlook on life. ~ Susan, mother of three

I'm now in the best shape and health of my life. I've always been an avid exerciser, but I took time off when I had my children. I wanted to get back into a routine, but I found that after taking 3 years off, it was really difficult to motivate myself. I knew I needed to do it, but I was always finding excuses for why I couldn't start. I saw an ad for a personal trainer in my neighborhood and I decided that I really needed to do this for myself. She initially gave me the push I needed, but once I started seeing results, it was easy to wake up every morning and find time to exercise. Results, weight loss, and improved health were the only motivations I needed. Now, on the days I don't exercise, I feel as though something is missing and that I didn't do everything I was supposed to. Exercise is an important part of my life now. ~ Kim, mother of two

The two things that make exercise work for me are convenience and fun. If a workout is not very easy to get to or to get done, it may not happen. Having equipment in my basement is the easiest for me right now as a stay-at-home mommy. But I have another one on the way and I feel like I may need to join a place with childcare once the baby is born. Right now, I can work out before my daughter gets up or after she goes to school, so I have tons of flexibility (that I haven't had for the past 5 years). In the earlier years, my daughter was a part of my workout. I carried her in the baby carrier as I did the elliptical glider when she was 0-1 year old, used the baby jogger routinely from 6 months on, walked to the park almost daily during nice weather (mommy gets some fun and baby gets some fun). But once she started fighting me about going for walks, I found it easier to join a gym with childcare. Then I really felt like I could focus completely on the workout, and I could work out in different ways that I couldn't do with my daughter, like swim or take spinning classes. But the gym HAS to be CONVENIENT. If it's too far away I'm not going to go! Plus it has to be FUN to me. Now I have a fantastic treadmill and I Tivo Oprah and watch it while I speed walk. What could be more fun than that? How could that ever not be enjoyable? If it's nice outside I walk through the neighborhood or on a trail and listen to tapes. I love it! I've found I do better if I get the workout in before I shower for the day. Once I shower I have much less of a tendency to want to get sweaty that day. ~ Beth, mother of one with a second child on the way

The reason I originally started to work out was because I was overweight and I wanted to look good again for me. Then I realized after I started working out that it wasn't just because of those reasons, but it was also because I am getting older and I wanted to make sure I was around to see my kids grow up and see them raise their families, and at that time my mom had so many health issues that I didn't want to end up like her. I also read and heard about some of the health issues that seem to appear when you hit the peri-menopause and menopausal stage of your life. I am trying to avoid having those issues as well. It is hard to continue to work out on a regular basis because I am a full-time mom with a full-time job and I get tired. But I think of those reasons above and that is why I do it. ~ Lori O., mother of three

I am motivated to exercise for many different reasons. Sometimes, it's a class that I like and I look forward to going to the gym. Sometimes it's just a matter of habit, and I go without really thinking about it. I also tell my children how important it is to exercise, and I insist that they participate in a sport of their choosing. So I feel it's important to exercise regularly as a good example to them, and to practice what I preach. Also, I exercise regularly because I don't like the way I look when I'm not exercising. Even if I haven't gained any weight from not exercising, I feel as though I look different. ~ *Lori T., mother of three*

I've placed roses in three places in my house — next to my bed for first thing in the morning — in the living room where I often decide not to exercise — in the kitchen where the food is. I love roses — they make me feel feminine and represent my true self to me . . . a visual reminder that I need to matter. On my way — making it happen — one choice at a time. ~ *Christi, mother of two*

I was not very sporty in my younger life but I loved dance and took ballet as a child. In college I was involved in the modern dance theatre and then after college, I did aerobic dance for many years, then step aerobics. Recently, I have taken up swimming as well since my kids are year round competitive swimmers and they inspire me! I exercise because I feel more energetic and less fatigued and have a better sense of well being. Also, my blood pressure and cholesterol levels are slightly high and I want to live as long as I can without taking medication. My kids are really active in sports. My husband and I want to keep up with them, as well as provide role models for my kids for being healthy. I swim twice a week with a masters class. We have a coach and most of the adults are very fast and nationally ranked. We work on sprints, distance, and technique. My plan is that I can always swim no matter what heath problems afflict me in old age so I want to improve my technique and stamina. It is much harder than step aerobics! I like the cross conditioning. My kids have inspired me — when I see them in meets swimming their hearts out I think, "I should be doing that too!" ~ Norma, mother of two

I am a new mom with an amazing 7-month old daughter, who also took an amazing toll on my body! Prior to getting pregnant with her, I had lost 80 pounds by changing my eating habits and walking. Walking was my only exercise (and occasional dancing on weekends — ohhh the life of a 21 year old!). I gained 80 lbs while pregnant since high protein foods and lots of walking weren't too appealing to me at the time. Now, 7 months later I am back to my plan and have lost 30 lbs. I like to take the time to take a walk every night (outside if possible). It is an amazing stress reliever, and a very healthy and low impact workout. Eventually I became addicted to it. Walking at night when the kids are settled down with a care taker or husband or possibly sleeping is great because it's cool outside, all your responsibilities are taken care of at home and it actually can help you get a better night's sleep. I wake up refreshed and on time every morning for the first time ever! ~ Elizabeth, mother of one

One of the reasons that I have been able to make weekly workouts a part of my life is because I see the results of my hard work. I look back to when I first started working out, and I could never imagine going back to the way that I was. I wish I had started this earlier in my life. Another reason that I am motivated to work out is because that is "my time" to do something great for my mind and body. Due to my constant busy schedule there is not much time left to devote to myself. This time is a great escape for me. That hour actually helps me to forget about everything else that I have going on and relieves the stress that I have built up. I feel as though I am better equipped to deal with the rest of the day. I guess you can say that working out is like therapy for me. I have come to rely upon it! ~ Shari, mother of two

Exercising gives me the opportunity to turn the "outside off" and the" inside on" for one hour a day so I can focus on myself and let the outside world go by. ~ Michele, mother of one

My husband and I realized the importance of health about a year and a half ago when my husband's mother was diagnosed with stomach cancer. It was a big wake-up call for all of us. Fortunately, she is a survivor and is doing very well. The experience helped us to realize that there are a lot of things that we cannot control but also a lot of things that we can control when it comes to health . . . like exercise and healthy eating. My husband and I have been exercising for over a year now. It's hard sometimes, especially with my husband since he comes home late. But he goes to the gym even late at night. Our bodies seem to crave it now. ~ Nancy, mother of two

My 10-year old English Springer Spaniel motivates me to exercise! She craves long hikes in the woods, so she gets me outside almost everyday, regardless of the weather. ~ Teresa, mother of twins

When I'm running, the refrain going through my mind is that the next hour will pass. At the end of it, do I want to have finished my training or have watched another TV show and eaten more than I need? The certainty of time passing keeps me moving every time. ~ Gloria, mother of one

I have struggled with my weight since I was a child but really felt the effects of a sedentary lifestyle in my early 30s. And I realized I have the metabolism of a hibernating bear! The only thing that helps me counter-balance those things and allows me to eat dessert once in a while (OK more than once in awhile) is exercise. Specifically, I now realize that I must do BOTH aerobic exercise and strength training. Sticking to it three times a week has allowed me to lose 26 pounds since the birth of my second son and I feel so much stronger and healthier overall. ~ Kay, mother of two

Sometimes when I want to exercise and I'm not in the mood, I trick myself and say that I'm just going to stretch. Then, as I start stretching, the next thing I know, I'm doing more than I planned! ~ Brenda, mother of one

More Words of Wisdom from Varied Sources

Visualization is a powerful thing. You must picture success — you have to be able to SEE it, feel it, and already be there in your mind. Live as if you are already there. Think as if you are already there.

The only thing that often separates successful people from non-successful people is ACTION.

There is no finish line. — Nike

Just do it. — Nike

My challenge to you is attitude. This is a long-term process. It's a choice, a priority, and a lifestyle. It's about forever. There is no finish line. It's all about making small changes little by little that you have no intention of ever stopping. They will slowly add up.

Exercise is one thing that cannot be delegated. Nobody can do this for you but you!

More may be better than less, but some is better than none.

Done is better than perfect, especially when perfect prevents actions.

What you focus on grows. Think positive always!

Recall that coaching is a profession that helps you find the part within you to accomplish more than you ever thought you could. Here are some phrases and analogies from my colleagues at Wellcoaches®:

When a baby learns to walk, they need a lot of help and fall a lot. We never scold them for falling or tell them to "forget it, they'll never get it." And so it is with exercise or any new endeavor. Why do we expect perfection from ourselves from day one?

A football team gains and loses yardage the whole game. They don't quit in the first quarter after losing yardage. Success is not measured in the short term, but in the long term. Keep working toward your goals!

Be wary of "cognitive quicksand" — the irrational or overly negative thinking that causes us to get stressed out and stop believing in ourselves. When you don't nip this in the bud, these negative thoughts drag you down and cause you to give up.

It's easier to act yourself into a new way of thinking than to think yourself into a new way of acting. No matter what it is — get started. You will feel better and be glad you did. If you wait around to feel motivated, you could be waiting a long time!

I've always liked the following story. I do not know the author or the origin. I received it through one of those chain emails and knew immediately that it was a keeper. I try to remember this story whenever I think I am filling my days with the wrong "stuff":

A philosophy professor stood before his class and had some items in front of him. When the class began, wordlessly he picked up a large empty mayonnaise jar and proceeded to fill it with rocks, rocks about 2" in diameter. He then asked the students if the jar was full. They agreed that it was. So the professor then picked up a box of pebbles and poured them into the jar. He shook the jar lightly. The pebbles, of course, rolled into the open areas between the rocks. He then asked the students again if the jar was full. They agreed it was. The students laughed. The professor picked up a box of sand and poured it into the jar. Of course, the sand filled up everything else.

"Now," said the professor, "I want you to recognize that this is your life. The rocks are the important things — your family, your partner, your health, and your children — things that if everything else was lost and only they remained, your life would still be full. The pebbles are the other things that matter like your job, your house, and your car. The sand is everything else, the small stuff.

If you put the sand into the jar first, there is no room for the pebbles or the rocks. The same goes for your life. If you spend all your time and energy on the small stuff, you will never have room for the things that are important to you. Pay attention to the things that are critical to your happiness. Play with your children. Take time to get medical checkups. Take your partner out dancing. There will always be time to go to work, clean the house, give a dinner party and fix the disposal. Take care of the rocks first — the things that really matter. Set your priorities. The rest is just sand."

Appendix 5

64 Reasons to Exercise!

1. Exercise burns 2–12 times as many calories per minute as sitting.
2. Exercise can help reduce the amount of fat on your body.
3. Exercise increases your muscle mass.
4. Exercise improves the strength and endurance of your existing muscle mass.
5. Exercise helps fight fatigue.
6. Exercise just makes you feel better!
7. Nobody else is going to do it for you.
8. Exercise gives you more energy.
9. Exercise gives you a more positive attitude.
10. Exercise gives you more confidence in your ability to accomplish goals.
11. Exercise success translates into mental fortitude for other challenges in life.
12. Exercise increases your body confidence.
13. Exercise improves your sex life.
14. Exercise reduces symptoms of PMS.
15. Exercise increases your bone density, decreasing your risk of osteoporosis.

16. Exercise lubricates your joints to supply more nutrients for healthier cartilage tissue.
17. Exercise can prevent constipation.
18. Exercise helps your body better regulate insulin and blood sugar levels.
19. Exercise reduces your risk of diabetes.
20. Exercise increases anti-inflammatory hormones, which may help prevent some forms of cancer.
21. Exercise reduces your risk of cardiovascular disease.
22. Exercise reduces high blood pressure.
23. Exercise can reduce total cholesterol.
24. Exercise can help increase HDL cholesterol (the good kind).
25. You've got to use it or lose it.
26. Exercise increases your resting metabolic rate.
27. Exercise increases your metabolic rate during all of your daily activities.
28. Exercise helps you perform the activities of daily life with less strain.
29. Exercise improves the flexibility of your muscles and joints.
30. Exercise helps improve your balance.
31. Exercise helps improve your posture.
32. Exercise helps reduce lower back pain.
33. Exercise improves your self-esteem.
34. Exercise reduces depression.
35. Exercise reduces anxiety.
36. Exercise reduces stress.
37. Exercise reduces absenteeism at work or school.
38. Exercise helps you spend less in health care costs.
39. Exercise helps you concentrate better.

40. Exercise helps you work more efficiently.
41. Exercise helps you sleep better.
42. Exercise makes your heart stronger.
43. Exercise makes your lungs stronger.
44. Exercise increases your cardiovascular endurance.
45. Exercise helps your clothes fit better.
46. Because your doctor wants you to!
47. Exercise enhances overall function of the brain and nerves.
48. Exercise helps keep you strong as you age.
49. Exercise promotes your independence as you age.
50. You'll always be able to carry in your own groceries.
51. Exercise helps you recover from surgery faster.
52. Exercise helps symptoms of arthritis (except during an acute inflammation).
53. Exercise strengthens your immune system, helping you fight off colds and flu.
54. Exercise helps you keep up with your kids.
55. Exercise helps your migraine headaches.
56. Exercise makes it easier to go up and down the stairs without getting out of breath.
57. Exercise eases lots of miscellaneous aches and pains.
58. Exercise is something you can do to have time for yourself.
59. Exercise gives you a natural high.
60. Exercise makes you want to eat healthier.
61. Exercise helps you feel young.
62. Exercise helps you feel like exercising some more!
63. Exercise helps you clear your head.
64. Exercise is a great way to do something for yourself that no one else can do!

Appendix 6

Resources for the Busy Mom

My Websites — Please come visit me!

www.busymomsolutions.com

Visit me at Busy Mom Solutions for even more resources and support tailored just for you, the busy mom who wants to be fit and healthy. Here are just a few of the things you'll find:

- Easy ordering for additional copies of *The Busy Mom's Ultimate Fitness Guide.*
- An exercise DVD that corresponds to the exercises recommended in this book.
- Fitness kits that you can order that contain pedometers, exercise balls, tubing, and more. You'll be able to get started right away with your new exercise plan!
- Free downloadable extras, such as a mini poster of the "64 Reasons to Exercise," a handy exercise log, and much more.
- Additional abdominal exercises and weight-training exercises when you're ready for more variety.
- An opportunity to connect with me and with other busy moms who are trying to make regular exercise a part of their lives. There will be group phone coaching sessions, teleseminars, and much more! Be sure to visit

and join the Busy Mom Solutions mailing list for great tips and to hear about the latest offerings.

- Motivational seminars and keynotes for your group or organization. Contact me for more information.

www.fitness-insight.com

Visit me at this site to find out more about my fitness and wellness business, Fitness InSight. I offer personal fitness training and metabolism testing to clients in the vicinity of Germantown, Maryland (Washington D.C. metropolitan area), and private wellness coaching via the telephone (for clients living anywhere!). On this site, you can sign up to receive my free monthly e-newsletter, *A Little Fitness InSight,* offering practical fitness and wellness tips that can make a difference in your daily life.

www.cathymoxley.com

Visit me here to find my online media kit, including a summary of my areas of expertise and bio, endorsements, downloadable high-resolution photos, and media experience. Members of the media are welcome to call or email to schedule interviews and appearances.

www.testyourmetabolism.com

Visit me at this site for information about my metabolism testing services in the Washington D.C. metropolitan area. You'll also find a link to search for providers of this service in your area. Finding out your resting metabolic rate gives you an accurate idea of how many calories your body burns each day so that you can plan how many calories you should eat to meet your goals. Metabolic exercise testing will tell you how many total calories and how many fat calories your body is burning per minute at different heart rate ranges while exercising.

Fabulous Organizations Related to Fitness and Wellness

Wellcoaches® (national provider and training organization for wellness coaching) www.wellcoaches.com

IDEA Health and Fitness Association: www.ideafit.com

The American Council on Exercise (ACE): www.acefitness.org

The American College of Sports Medicine (ACSM): www.acsm.org

New Leaf Health and Fitness (metabolism testing technology and provider locator): www.newleaffitness.com

The National Weight Loss Registry: www.nwcr.ws

The National Strength and Conditioning Association: www.nsca-lift.org

Fitness Programs for Moms

The following fitness programs and networks are tailored specifically for moms. Visit their websites to see if their services and locations are a good fit for you.

www.babybootcamp.com
www.healthymomsfitness.com
www.seemommyrun.com
www.strollerfit.com
www.strollerstrides.com
www.strollercize.com

Resources on Being More Active

www.americaonthemove.org
www.shapeup.org

Recommended Reading

The Ultimate Weight Solution: The 7 Keys to Weight Loss Freedom (Free Press 2003) Dr. Phil McGraw.

Unclutter Your Life (Golden Lakes Publishing Co., Inc. 2004) Jenny Lovins, www.unclutteryourlifetoday.com

Squeezing Your Size 14 Self into A Size 6 World: A Real Woman's Guide to Food, Fitness, and Self-Acceptance (Champion Press Ltd., 2004) Carrie Myers Smith, www.championpress.com/books/squeeze.htm.

Bibliography

1. American College of Sports Medicine. *ACSM's Guidelines for Exercise Testing and Prescription,* Seventh Edition, 2006. Philadelphia, PA: Lippincott Williams & Wilkins.
2. American College of Obstetrics and Gynocology (ACOG). *Exercise During Pregnancy and the Postpartum Period* (ACOG Committee Opinion: Number 267, January 2002)
3. Evolve Sports Medicine Group, *Metabolic Physiology,* 2004.
4. Prochaska, James O. *Changing for Good: A Revolutionary Six-Stage Program for Overcoming Bad Habits and Moving Your Life Positively Forward,* New York, NY: Avon Books, 1994.
5. Prochaska, James O. "Enhancing Motivation to Change." In B.B. Wilford, A.W. Graham, & T.K. Schultz (Eds.), *Principles of Addictive Medicine* (Third Edition). 825–838 Chevy Chase, MD: American Society of Addictive Medicine.
6. Watkins, Sheila S. *Healthy Moms Perinatal Fitness Instructor Training Manual,* 1999.
7. Wellcoaches Corporation, *Wellcoaches Fitness Coaching Skills Manual,* 2003

About the Author

Cathy Moxley has been helping people get fit, lose weight, and stay motivated since 1987. She specializes in helping busy moms make sense of an endless sea of health information, put together a plan that will work, and find that part within them that will keep it going! She focuses on teaching practical fitness, nutrition, and wellness information that is easy to understand and apply to your busy daily life.

She founded Fitness InSight in 1996 with just a few personal training clients in her home gym. Today, her business has grown to include motivational seminars, coaching, metabolism assessment, managing her four websites, and of course, writing.

Her degrees include a Master of Arts in Exercise Physiology, and a Bachelor of Science degree in Kinesiological Sciences, both from the University of Maryland. She holds certifications from the National Strength and Conditioning Association (N.S.C.A.), the American Council on Exercise (A.C.E.), Healthy Moms®, and Wellcoaches®.

She and her husband John, and their three children, Jenna, Jeff, and Matthew, live in Germantown, Maryland. When she is not helping clients or writing, she spends a good deal of time making peanut butter and jelly sandwiches and shuttling kids to soccer, swimming, and preschool. Life is good!

The Busy Mom's Ultimate Fitness Guide
Get Motivated and Find the Solution that Works for You!

ORDER FORM

❐ YES! I'd like to order a copy of
The Busy Mom's Ultimate Fitness Guide.

Online: Go to www.busymomsolutions.com (credit card orders only)

Fax: Fax this form to: 301-576-4420 (credit card orders only)

Mail: Send this form with check or credit card information to:

Fitness InSight
13402 Queenstown Lane
Germantown, MD 20874

Name: ____

Address: ____

City: ______________________ State: _____ Zip: ____________

Telephone: ____

Email Address: _____________________________________

Quantity: _____ Price per book: $ 19.95 Book Total: ____________
Sales Tax:* ____________
Shipping: $ 3.85 for the first book ____________
$ 2.00 for each additional book ____________
Total Enclosed: ____________

*Please add 5% sales tax for books shipped to Maryland addresses.

Payment Method:
❐ Check (made payable to: Fitness InSight)
❐ Credit Card ___ Visa ___ MasterCard

Card Number: ______________________________________

Name on Card ____________________ Exp. Date: ____________

Signature: ____

Questions? Leave a voice message at 301-576-4420
or email orders@fitness-insight.com